Other Books by Ann Tam

The Poop Book For Pets: Clues to your Pet's Health

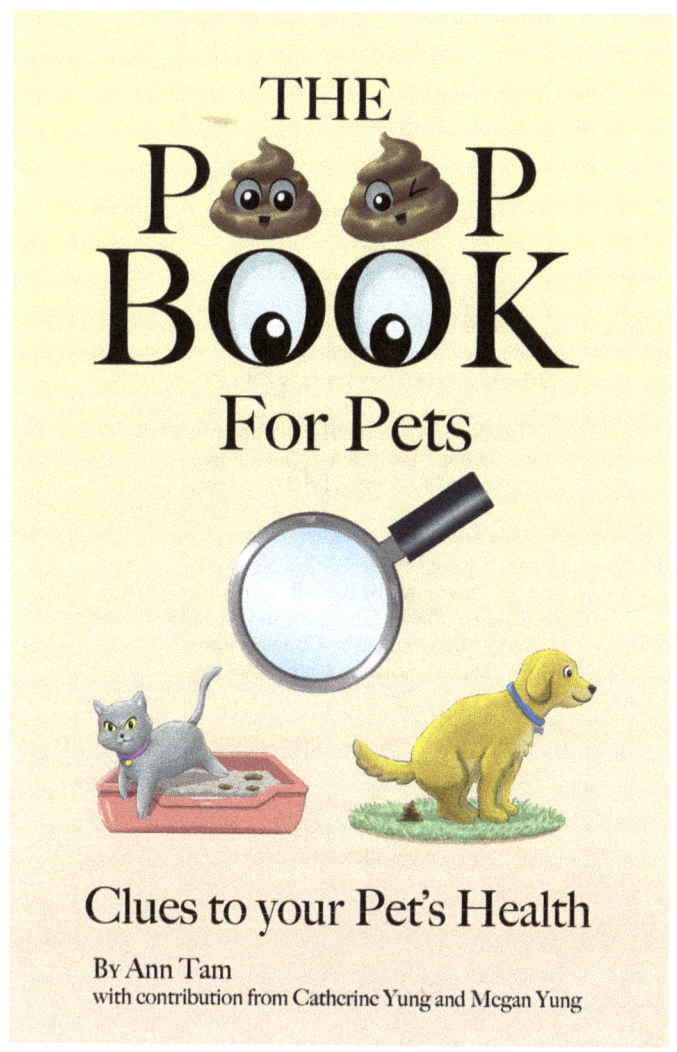

Visit Ann Tam at Sikieherbs.com

Copyright © 2025 by Ann Tam

All rights reserved.

No portion of this book may be reproduced in any form or by any means, electronic or mechanical, including photocopying, recording, or by any information storage and retrieval system now known or hereafter invented, without prior written permission from the publisher, except for brief quotations used in reviews, articles, or scholarly work.

ISBN 979-8-9989641-2-1 (Paperback)
ISBN 979-8-9989641-3-8 (eBook)
ISBN 979-8-9989641-5-2 (Hardcover)

Edited by Dr. Patricia Nguyen
Illustrated by Russell Gunning
Cover design by Walter Lundquist and Russell Gunning
Cover Edited by Connie Tam
Interior design by Catherine Yung

First Edition

Published by Ann Tam / Silkie LLC
Printed in the United States of America
www.silkieherbs.com

Stay Connected

"If you found this book helpful, please consider leaving a review. Your feedback not only supports our mission but also helps others discover the power of natural healing and Traditional Chinese Medicine.

Thank you for honoring time-tested wisdom and choosing a natural path to health. Every poop tells a story, and true healing begins with paying attention to the body's signals.

Health is wealth. Take care of your body — it's the only place you have to live. Even small changes in your stool can reveal big insights about your well-being."

Disclaimer

The information provided in this book on different types of stools is intended for general educational and informational purposes only. It is not a substitute for professional medical advice, diagnosis, or treatment. The content within this book is based on general observations and may not cover all possible variations or individual circumstances.

While efforts have been made to ensure the accuracy and completeness of the information, the authors and publisher make no representations or warranties of any kind, express or implied, about the reliability, suitability, or availability of the information contained within this book.

Readers are strongly advised to consult with qualified healthcare professionals for personalized advice and guidance related to their specific health conditions. Stool characteristics can vary widely between individuals, and changes in stool appearance may indicate various health issues.

Medical knowledge is subject to ongoing research and development, and the information in this book may not reflect the most current medical understanding. The authors and publisher disclaim any liability for any direct or indirect consequences resulting from the use of the information presented in this book.

This book does not endorse or recommend specific medical treatments, and any reference to particular stool characteristics should not be considered as a diagnosis or medical recommendation. It is essential for readers to seek professional medical evaluation and guidance for any concerns related to their digestive health.

The reader is responsible for their own health decisions, and the authors and publisher are not liable for any actions or decisions made based on the information provided in this book.

By reading this book, the reader acknowledges and agrees to the terms of this disclaimer.

Acknowledgements

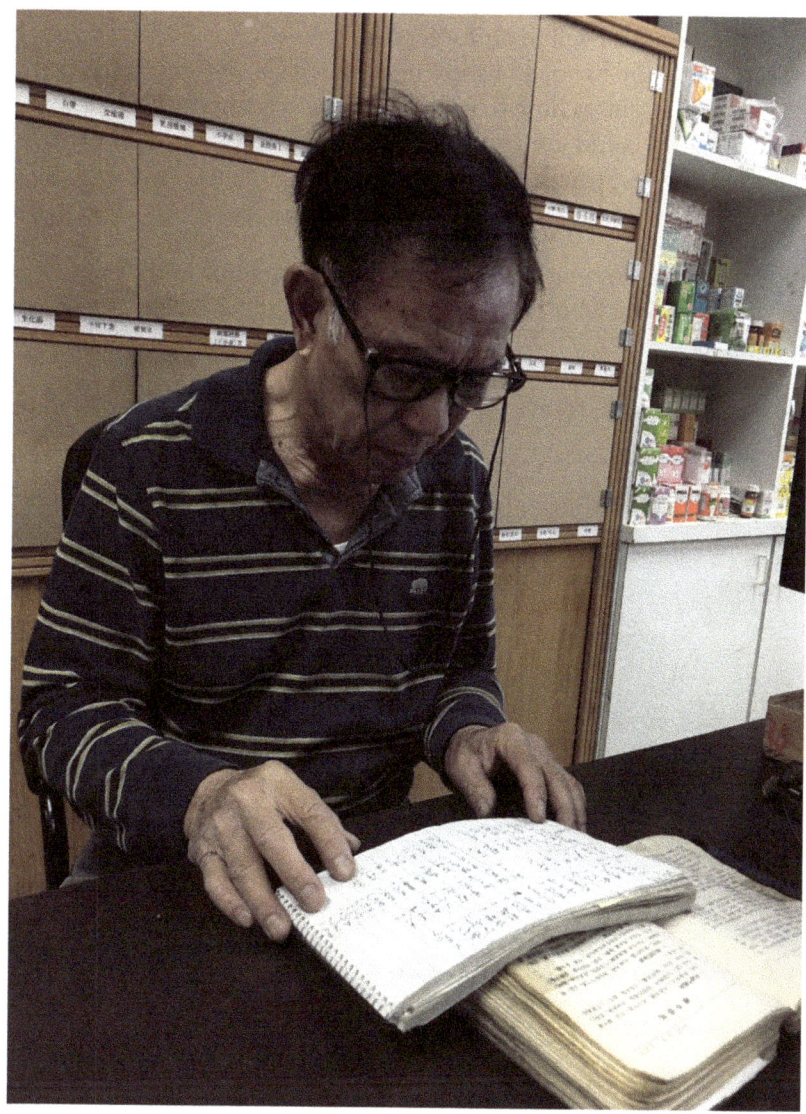

This book is dedicated to my father, Hon Dam, the fourth-generation herbalist of our family and the heart behind Silkie Herbs.

Dad, you taught me everything that cannot be found in textbooks — the art of real-life diagnosis, what to look for, and how to trust both my eyes and my instincts. You showed me how to listen to the body's hidden language, not only through pulse and tongue, but through the many subtle clues that guide true healing.

I still remember those days when we traveled together, backpacks on our shoulders, riding trains across China, filled with cigarette smoke that lingered in the beds, the walls, and the air we breathed. We searched for herb farmland, spoke with farmers, and studied pills and machines — plant by plant, formula by formula — laying the foundation for what later became Silkie. Those journeys were uncomfortable at times, but I carry them now as treasures, memories of lessons you gave me not just in medicine, but in perseverance, sacrifice, and love.

I studied alongside you as you explored how to use modern machines to support our traditional ways of making honey pills. Together, we learned how to balance ancient methods with modern technology, from pill-making to testing in the lab, ensuring that every formula met the highest standard of safety and quality. You showed me how tradition and science could work hand in hand, and those lessons remain at the core of Silkie Herbs today.

But more than the machines or the labs, I will never forget the times you worked with your hands. I can still see you making honey pills from scratch, all by hand, and showing us each careful step in the process. I can still hear you singing the old herb songs as you taught us how to prepare and process herbs in the most traditional way, passing down knowledge that no classroom could ever capture. And I can still picture your strong hands cutting herbs with the ancestral knife passed down through generations, showing us not only the skill of preparation but also the weight of heritage in every cut.

I cannot thank you enough for saving my child and myself. Because of your knowledge, your persistence, and your faith in the healing power of Traditional Chinese Medicine, my daughter Catherine can live like a normal kid today. That gift will never be forgotten.

Dad, I love you, and I will remember you forever. This book, and all my work, carries your spirit forward.

— Ann

Contents

Preface	IX
Introduction	XI
The Significance of Bowel Movements	1
The Fascinating Adventure from Food to Poop	3
What's Considered a Normal Poop and Frequency?	7
Understanding the Different types of Stool Odors	13
Understanding the Different Colors of Stools	15
Understanding Stool Types	25
Bumpy, Lumpy Stool	
Dry, Dark Brown Stool with Cracks	33
Initial Dry and Hard Segment, Then Soft and Thinner Stool	37
Finger-Like Stool Pieces	43
Fluffy Stool Pieces that are Mushy, Loose, or Soft	51
Stool With White Dots or Thin White Worms	57
Soft Blobs Of Stool That Require Some Straining To Pass	63
Floating Stool	71
Sinking & Sticky Stool	77
Dry, Hard, Dark Pebbles That Are Hard To Pass	81
Dark To Light Watery Stool Multiple Times Within A Day With Rotten Odor	87
Dark Yellow, Watery Stool With or Without Foul Odor	93
Light Yellow, Watery Stool With or Without a Foul "Fishy" Odor	97
Green Stool	103
Pale Stool	107

Blood in The Stool With Or Without Pus And Mucus	113
Black Tar-Like Or Dark Purple Bloody Stool	119
Bright Red Blood	125
Exploring Fecal Incontinence Causes	131
Understanding the Different Types of Constipation and What Causes Them	133
Lactose Intolerance in Traditional Chinese Medicine	137
TCM Perspective on Common Gut Health Practices & Mistakes	139
Diet and Lifestyle Tips for Healthy Bowel Movements	141
Seeking Professional Guidance	143
Conclusion: Your Poop, Your Health Story	145
TCM Digestive Pattern Quick Guide	147
Food & Poop Matching Guide	149
TCM Stool Types & Herbs Guide	151
Stool Tracker	157
Index	159

Preface

This book was born out of the countless times patients looked at me with a mix of confusion, embarrassment, or the distinct expression of *"Did you really just ask me that?"* — when I inquired about their poop. Their faces, in various shades of protest, seemed to say, *"But I'm not here for anything digestive!"* Fair enough — but in Chinese Medicine, we look at the *whole* picture. And yes, that includes what's going on in the bathroom.

You see, Chinese Medicine practitioners piece together patterns from a variety of symptoms — some obvious, some surprisingly subtle. Poop just happens to be one of those clues that can say a lot (sometimes more than you wanted to know) about what's going on internally. It helps us confirm diagnoses alongside other time-honored methods like tongue reading, pulse taking, and abdominal palpation.

Between the two of us — Ann Tam and me — we've clocked over 20 years of clinical experience. It's almost comical to realize I've spent the last decade talking about poop professionally and still find it fascinating. Ann, on the other hand, has been around poop talk since before she could walk. She hails from a long and deeply rooted line of Chinese herbalists, and let me tell you — she is the most brilliant Master Herbalist I know (and I know a few!).

I consider myself incredibly lucky to have met Ann — not just because she's a 5th-generation herbalist with wisdom that could fill volumes — but because she's got a sharp eye for patterns and an unwavering passion for sharing Chinese Medicine with others. She's also the tireless force behind the depth and thoroughness of this book. Five generations' worth of herbal knowledge? That's some serious ancestral Google.

Our hope is that this book helps normalize the often-taboo topic of poop, and maybe even makes it a little less awkward to talk about (we promise, it gets easier). We want this book to be a bridge — one that connects curious patients, passionate students, and fellow practitioners to the rich, nuanced world of Chinese Medicine.

Whether you're reading this on a quest for better health, or because you're a healthcare professional looking to deepen your understanding, we hope you find it insightful, accessible, and — dare we say — enjoyable. We certainly enjoyed writing it, one conversation about poop at a time.

Patricia Nguyen
San Diego, CA
Summer 2025

Introduction

Over the years, I've lost track of how many times I've asked patients about their poop and heard the same confident answer: *"Oh, my poop is normal."*

But when I start asking for details — the color, the shape, the texture — or when they're brave enough to show me a photo, it often turns out their "normal" isn't actually normal at all. Many people don't realize how far from healthy their digestion has drifted, simply because they've never been taught what truly healthy poop should look like or how often they should go each day.

It's not just patients, either. When I teach acupuncture students, I'm still surprised by how often they underestimate the value of stool in diagnosis. Without clear visual references or a solid understanding of what each variation means, it's easy to miss how much these subtle changes reveal about the body's internal balance — or imbalance. That's what inspired me to write this book.

I grew up immersed in this knowledge. As a fifth-generation herbalist, I learned early on that poop isn't just waste — it's a health report. My father, a master herbalist, taught me that the body speaks through many signs, and stool is one of the most honest. It never lies, and it often tells the story of what's happening inside before any other symptom appears.

In this book, I've organized the content to take you on a clear journey. We begin with what normal, healthy poop looks like, then move step by step through different patterns of imbalance. Sometimes these stages overlap, especially during illness, when changes in diet can create a mix of stool types. For each type, you'll find an explanation of the underlying causes from a Traditional Chinese Medicine perspective, and you'll see how those patterns connect to the body's systems such as the Liver, Spleen, Kidneys, Blood, and Qi.

A note on terminology: you'll notice that certain words are capitalized. In TCM, terms like "Liver" or "Spleen" refer to an entire functional system, not just the physical organ recognized in Western medicine. The Liver in TCM, for example, is not just a physical organ that filters toxins, but a whole network that regulates the smooth flow of Qi and Blood, influences emotions, and affects digestion. When you see a capitalized term, it is referring to the TCM system and its broader role in health, rather than the anatomical organ alone.

Each poop type in this book is paired with a description of symptoms to help you identify the pattern in your own body, an explanation of the underlying causes, recommendations for what foods to eat and what to avoid, and lifestyle tips to support recovery. For quick reference, I have included short TCM notes under each illustration, and the illustrations themselves are designed to be clear and educational without being graphic or uncomfortable. I've also added background sections that explain the vital roles of Qi, Blood, and the major organ systems, since these foundations keep us strong, balanced, and resilient.

You'll probably notice some repetition as you read. Many of the dietary recommendations are similar, since greasy, processed, or overly cold foods tend to weaken digestion in general. Likewise, emotions such as irritation, frustration, or anger can appear across multiple imbalances because health rarely breaks down in isolation. And organ systems like the Spleen, Liver, and Kidneys are often described as "powerhouses" in TCM because of their central importance in maintaining overall balance. This overlap is intentional. It reflects the way the body really works — interconnected, layered, and dynamic. Think of it less as redundancy and more as reinforcement, showing you how the same threads weave through many different health concerns.

To make this book especially practical, it has been designed in a larger format. This gives you space for clear illustrations, easy-to-read explanations, and a layout that works like a true reference guide. I've also included an Index at the back, so you can quickly look up specific symptoms, or organ systems without needing to flip through every chapter. Think of this as both a guide you can read cover to cover and a manual you can return to whenever you need clarity.

Along the way, we'll also address misleading diet trends and one-size-fits-all health advice that circulate online. These may seem harmless, but they can delay recovery, weaken the body further, and make it harder to correct imbalances. When you understand what your stool is telling you and respond appropriately, you gain the power to address small issues before they become bigger ones.

Aging is natural, but premature aging is avoidable. Once we know how to identify and address health issues early — sometimes just by looking at our poop — we can protect our vitality, slow down the aging process, and enjoy a healthier, more energetic life.

This book is meant to be both a guide and a reference. You can read it straight through to understand the full picture, or you can flip directly to the sections that match your current symptoms. Either way, you'll come away with practical tools you can use every day.

Health is wealth. Stay grounded, stay informed, and take care of your body — it's the only place you truly live.

Ann Tam
Westminster, CA
Summer 2025

The Significance of Bowel Movements

Bowel movement, often referred to as the act of pooping, is one of our body's chief methods of expelling waste and toxins. Similar to a house needing routine cleaning to remain livable, our bodies require consistent waste elimination to maintain good health. The nature of your stool offers insights into your diet, your body's processing efficiency, and, by extension, your overall health. Observing your stool before flushing can be an enlightening habit. So don't rush to flush.

Here are some key aspects to pay attention to when observing your bowel movements and what they can potentially reveal about your digestive health:

Color: The color of your poop can be a revealing sign. While brown poop is generally considered normal, a deviation from this color can signify different things. For example, green poop may indicate a high intake of leafy green vegetables. Black stool could suggest the possibility of internal bleeding. White stool might point to potential Liver-related issues. Because color can indicate problems with the digestive system, it is important to pay attention to the color of your stool.

Consistency: Healthy poop should be firm and easy to pass. A deviation from this can signify your digestive system is off. For example, hard or lumpy stool could indicate a lack of fluid or too much internal heat, potentially leading to constipation. Watery or loose stool could be a sign of too much internal cold, toxins, or food poisoning, potentially leading to diarrhea. The consistency of stools gives insight into the balance of heat and fluids in your body.

Shape: Ideally, your poop should have a smooth and cylindrical shape. Any other shape could indicate a potential issue within your digestive tract: Narrow ribbon-like poop could indicate obstruction of the large intestine. Mushy, mashed potato-like poop could indicate too much mucus in the digestive tract from eating too much dairy products, sweets, or cold foods and drinks. Hard and pebble-like poop could indicate too much heat stemming from excessive intake of hot natured items such as fried, grilled, or spicy foods; not drinking enough water; or prolonged Blood Deficiency and Dryness.

In this book, we use the term "mucus" to encompass the Traditional Chinese Medicine (TCM) terms "damp" and "phlegm" which refer to any pathological accumulation of moisture, fluids, or substances that may or may not be expelled from the body. For example, phlegm from the Lungs, runny nose, sinus congestion, lipoma, cyst, pus, excessive body fat, cholesterol, and inflammation are all forms of mucus.

The term "Blood Deficiency" in TCM means the body's supply of Blood does not meet the daily demand for Blood. Anemia is a form of Blood Deficiency, but not all Blood Deficiency patterns present with anemia. "Blood Deficiency and Dryness" is a pattern that presents when Blood Deficiency is long standing or chronic.

Frequency: A daily bowel movement, preferably in the morning, is often considered a sign of a healthy digestive system. Deviations from this norm, such as more frequent or less frequent movements, provide insight into how well your body absorbs nutrients from food and eliminates waste.

Poop Type	Possible Imbalance
Dark, hard, & dry	Excessive heat and a lack of fluids (too much Yang)
Dark, hard, dry, & pebbly	Blood & Qi Deficiency with dryness (lack of Yin & Yang)
Mushy, soft, sticky	Excess mucus or phlegm (lack of Yang or excess Yin)
Loose with undigested food	Food Retention or Food Poison (lack of Qi)
Watery with pain	Excess cold dampness or heat dampness (too much Yin or Yang)
Initially hard, then soft	Qi Deficiency with mucus (lack of Yang)

The table shows the imbalances linked to different stool types.

In the realm of TCM, practitioners closely examine these details because they offer clues about your overall health and the balance of Yin and Yang, as well as Blood and Qi (pronounced "chee") within your body.

In Chinese philosophy, Yin and Yang represent two complementary forces that influence various aspects of life, including health. Yin is associated with the moon and embodies qualities like cold and darkness, while Yang is associated with the sun and represents qualities such as heat and light. Maintaining a harmonious balance between these forces is essential for good health.

Blood serves as the vital fluid that nourishes the body, while Qi is the energy that flows throughout your body. When Blood and Qi are abundant and free-flowing, your body functions optimally. However, shortages or blockages of Blood and Qi can lead to health problems.

Your bowel movements hold a wealth of information about your diet, lifestyle, and health. This information guides TCM physicians in making dietary recommendations, prescribing appropriate herbal treatments, and selecting acupuncture points for treatment. So, let's delve even deeper into the formation of stool and explore its profound significance in maintaining overall health.

The Fascinating Adventure from Food to Poop

Let's embark on a journey through your body to discover how the food you eat undergoes a magical transformation into the waste known as poop. This journey involves a series of remarkable steps that work together like a well-orchestrated symphony.

The Mouth: Where It All Begins

Our adventure begins in the mouth, where the food you eat goes through both physical and chemical transformations. Think of your mouth as a portal to a grand stage of digestion. Physically, your food is broken down into smaller, manageable pieces as you chew it. Meanwhile, the chemical aspect starts with saliva, a fluid in your mouth that moistens the food and contains enzymes. These enzymes are like little workers that begin the process of breaking down carbohydrates in your food. This is why it's important to chew your food thoroughly and savor every bite.

The Esophagus: The Food Slide

After swallowing your chewed food, it embarks on a journey down the esophagus, a muscular tube that acts like a slide, guiding food down to your stomach. It's not just a passive slide; there's a wave-like muscle movement called peristalsis that ensures your food moves smoothly. However, sometimes, stomach acid can move in the wrong direction, causing a sensation known as acid reflux, which is quite uncomfortable.

The Stomach: The Food Processor

Your food's next destination is the stomach, which can be compared to a powerful food processor bowl. Here, your food is mixed with stomach acid and enzymes. Stomach acid serves a dual purpose: it helps to eliminate harmful bacteria in your food and assists in breaking down your food further. There are specialized enzymes in the stomach that focus on digesting proteins. While in this acidic environment, your food spends some quality time getting digested. However, it's worth noting that issues like gastric ulcers and hiatal hernias can disrupt this delicate balance.

The Spleen: The Powerhouse of Digestion (TCM Perspective)

In Traditional Chinese Medicine (TCM), the Spleen plays a vital role in digestion and overall vitality. Unlike its function in Western medicine as a blood-filtering organ, TCM sees the Spleen as the powerhouse of digestion, responsible for extracting nutrients from food and transforming them into Qi (vital energy), Blood, body fluids. Once food and liquids enter the body, the Spleen separates the pure essence, sending it upward to the Lungs and Heart to be distributed as nourishment, while the stomach directs residual food and nutrients downward. This delicate balance between ascending and descending functions maintains harmony in the digestive system.

When the Spleen functions optimally, the body thrives with strong digestion, abundant energy, and stable circulation. However, if the Spleen is weak or imbalanced, it can lead to poor digestion, bloating, fatigue, diarrhea, or fluid retention. Additionally, because the Spleen governs blood circulation, a deficiency in Spleen Qi can cause blood to escape its normal pathways, leading to symptoms like bruising, excessive menstrual bleeding, blood in the stool, or blood in the urine. Maintaining a healthy Spleen through proper diet and lifestyle choices ensures a steady flow of energy and nourishment throughout the body.

The Small Intestine: The Nutrient Extractor

In Traditional Chinese Medicine (TCM), the Small Intestine, a long coiled organ about 20 feet in adults, isn't just a digestive organ — it's a discerning sorter. After the Stomach has initially "fermented and ripened" the food, the Small Intestine receives this partially digested material and continues the process of separation. Its main function is to distinguish the "clear" (pure, essential nutrients and fluids) from the "turbid" (impure waste).

The clear part is sent upward to the Spleen, which then transports and transforms these vital substances into Qi and Blood to nourish the body. The turbid portion is sent downward: the solid waste to the Large Intestine for elimination, and excess fluids to the Bladder for transformation into urine.

In Western terms, the Small Intestine absorbs nutrients, while in TCM, it ensures proper sorting, assimilation, and elimination. When the Small Intestine is out of balance, it may result in abdominal discomfort, bloating, scanty or painful urination (dysuria), or irregular bowel movements. This organ's ability to effectively "separate the clear from the turbid" is essential for maintaining harmony between the digestive and urinary systems.

The Large Intestine: The Final Stop Before Poop

From the Small Intestine, digested food material continues onward and enters the Large Intestine, which is about 5 feet long in adults. The main role of the Large Intestine is to extract water from the remaining food material, gradually turning it into the familiar substance we call poop. This part of the journey involves the cecum, the colon, the rectum, and the anus. Your Large Intestine serves as a storage facility for poop until it's ready for elimination. As a storage that holds waste until it can be eliminated, the Large Intestine is prone to various disorders, including diverticulitis, Crohn's disease, colon cancer, and incontinence.

Accessory Organs of Digestion: The Backup Crew

In addition to the main players, we have supporting organs behind the scenes.

Pancreas: This gland produces enzymes crucial for breaking down carbohydrates, proteins, and fats. It also plays a pivotal role in regulating blood sugar levels by producing insulin. In TCM, the pancreas is considered a part of the Spleen.

Liver: The Liver is like a multitasking powerhouse. It stores energy in the form of glycogen, produces bile to help digest fats, and neutralizes toxins to help detoxify and purify the blood.

In addition to these functions, the Liver is responsible for promoting flow and movement throughout the body. By ensuring the smooth circulation of Qi, Blood, and body fluids, it helps maintain overall balance and harmony. The Liver's "flowing and spreading" function has three key aspects:

Regulating Qi – Ensuring the smooth flow of energy throughout the body.

Regulating emotions – Preventing emotional and mood imbalances like anger, frustration, and depression due to Qi stagnation.

Enhancing the digestive properties of the Spleen – Supporting digestion by promoting the proper movement of nutrients and waste.

Gallbladder: A small sac-like organ, the Gallbladder stores bile. When you eat, it contracts and releases bile into the Small Intestine to aid in the digestion of fats.

The Symphony of Digestion

The entire digestive process is like a grand orchestra, with each organ playing a unique role. The goal is to break food into essential nutrients that fuel your body for energy, growth, and repair. In TCM, proper digestion ensures the production of Qi, Blood, and fluids necessary for overall health.

How Long Does Digestion Take? Now, let's look into the timeline of food digestion and elimination. Consider a typical meal consisting of meat, vegetables, and grains.

After you chew and swallow your food, it stays in the Stomach for approximately 40 minutes to 6 hours, with an average of about 3 hours. From the Stomach, your food moves into the Small Intestine, where it can take anywhere from 2 to 7 hours to traverse the entire 20-foot length. The last stop is the Large Intestine. This is where poop starts to take shape. It takes a minimum of 10 hours to travel the 5-foot length of the Large Intestine before it's ready for elimination.

The exact timing can vary significantly from person to person, depending on several factors. Different foods have varying digestion times, with meats generally taking longer to digest than vegetables. Older adults typically experience slower digestion compared to younger individuals. Additionally digestive problems can either speed up or slow down the time it takes for digestion. Therefore, type of food intake, age and health of the individual will determine the total time from food consumption to poop elimination.

To maintain healthy bowel movements and support a smooth digestive process, consider these practical tips:

Eat a balanced diet. Consume a varied diet that includes plenty of vegetables, some meat, and a moderate amount of whole grains.

Eat at regular times. Establish consistent meal times, such as 7 a.m., 12 p.m., and 5 p.m. This creates a regular routine for your digestive system.

Chew thoroughly. Take your time to chew your food slowly and thoroughly to aid in the digestion process.

Stay hydrated. Ensure you drink an adequate amount of fluids at room temperature to support digestion.

Exercise daily. Include daily physical activity in your routine, such as walking with deep breathing for 15-60 minutes.

Listen to your body. Pay close attention to your body's signals and respond when you feel the urge to use the restroom. If you feel the urge, visit the bathroom as soon as possible. Avoid straining during bowel movements to maintain good digestive health.

By understanding this incredible journey from food to poop and following these practical tips, you can promote healthy digestion and maintain regular bowel movements to ensure your body functions optimally.

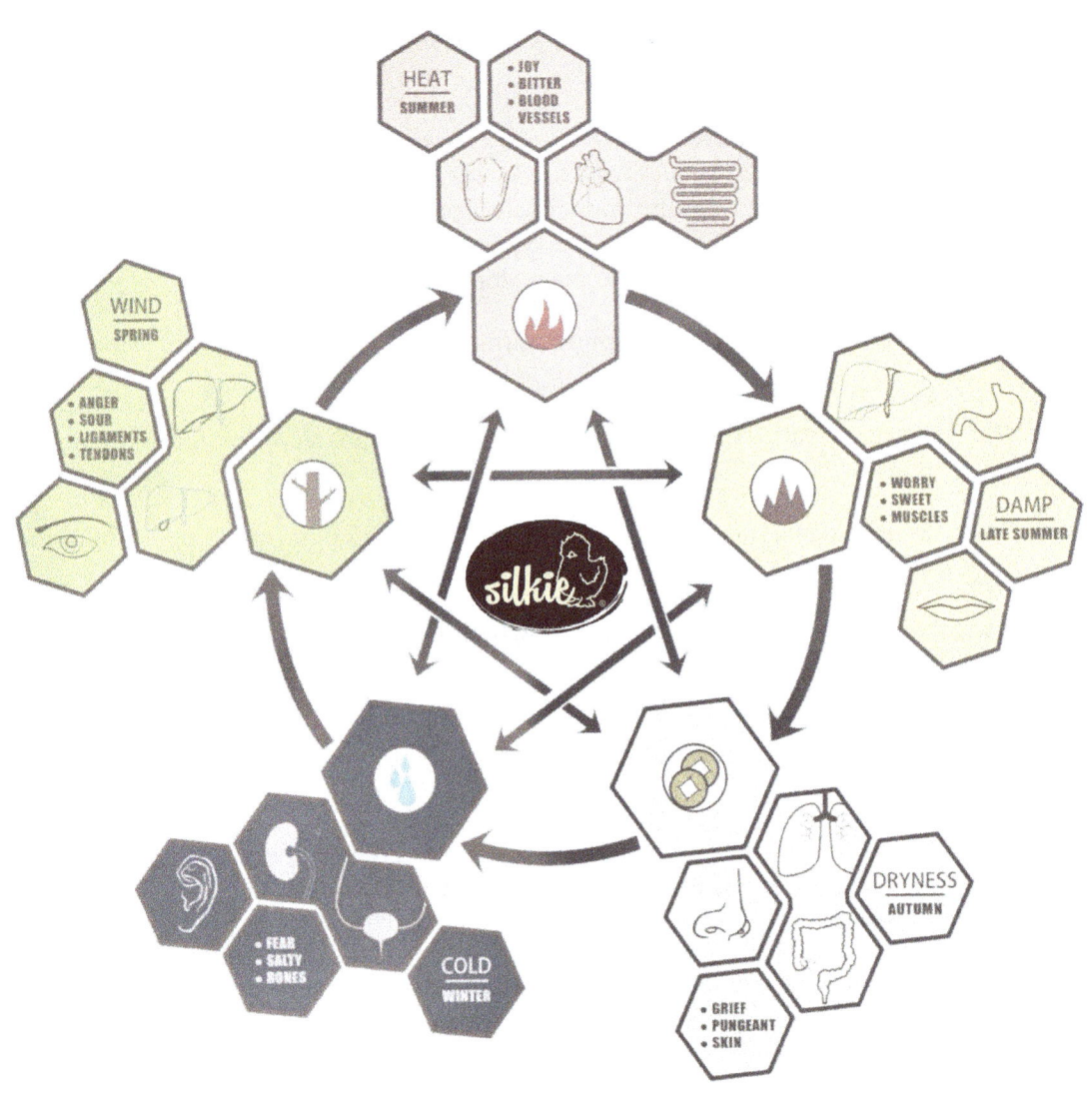

What's Considered a Normal Poop and Frequency?

How Often Should You Poop? What Your Bathroom Habits Say About Your Health

In this chapter, we'll take a closer look at how often you should be making trips to the bathroom and what the quality of your bowel movements reveals about your overall health. It might seem like an everyday, even awkward topic, but in Traditional Chinese Medicine (TCM) — and even in modern medicine—your poop is a vital sign of what's going on inside your body.

The Frequency of Pooping: What's Normal?

For someone with a well-functioning digestive system, the entire process — from eating food to digesting, absorbing nutrients, and finally eliminating waste — should take about 24 hours. In TCM, this is considered a smooth and balanced digestive rhythm. When everything is in harmony, you should pass one complete and satisfying bowel movement per day, ideally in the morning.

However, many people fall outside this rhythm, which can be an early signal that something is off in the body's internal balance.

If You Poop Several Times a Day...

Needing to go to the bathroom two, three, or more times daily — especially if the stool is loose or watery — may suggest that food is moving too quickly through your digestive system. In TCM, this can mean that the Spleen and Stomach Qi are weak, making it difficult to transform food into usable energy (Qi), Blood, and Body Fluids.

Because digestion is rushed, your body doesn't have enough time to properly absorb nutrients. This can eventually lead to deficiency-type symptoms like: fatigue, weak muscles, pale complexion, cold limbs, loose stools with undigested food. Over time, frequent or urgent bowel movements may deplete the body's energy reserves and lead to chronic imbalances, especially if left unaddressed.

If You Poop Only Once Every Few Days...

Going days without a bowel movement means your body is holding onto waste longer than it should. In TCM, this prolonged retention is often linked to patterns of heat accumulation, dryness, or Qi stagnation.

When waste lingers in the body, heat and toxins can accumulate and present externally as bad breath, acne, or skin rashes. Prolonged constipation can also affect your mood with increased irritability and alter your energy level. Sometimes, the cause may be a lack of fluids or blood (Dryness), an overconsumption of heating foods (like fried or spicy dishes), or emotional stress that disrupts the natural flow of Qi in the Large Intestine.

The Best Time to Poop, According to TCM

TCM teaches that the body follows a 24-hour circadian wellness clock, with each internal organ taking turns being most active. This system, called the Organ Clock, divides the day into twelve two-hour blocks, with each organ's energy peaking during its designated time.

Between 5 a.m. and 7 a.m., the Large Intestine is at its strongest. This is when your body is naturally preparing to eliminate waste from the previous day. The Yang energy of the sun begins to rise, waking the body up and stimulating digestion. This is why, in TCM, the ideal time to have a bowel movement is early in the morning, shortly after waking.

If you wake up and have a full, easy, and satisfying bowel movement without needing to rush or strain, it's a strong indicator that your digestion, energy flow, and organ systems are in balance.

24hr Wellness Wheel

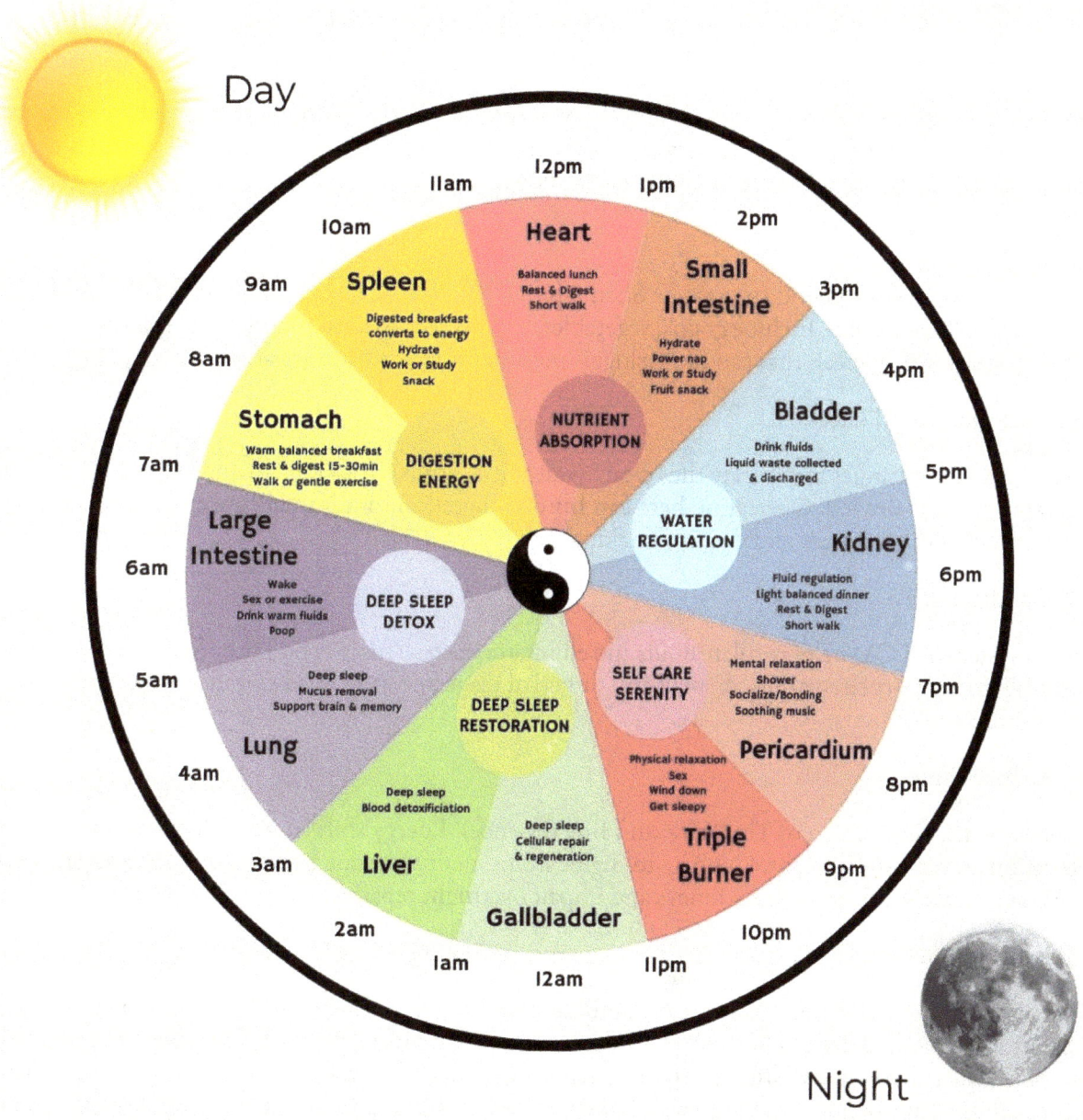

TCM, has long recognized that the body operates according to a natural rhythm — a 24-hour cycle in which each internal organ takes turns being most active. This concept is known as the Organ Clock or Horary Cycle. According to this ancient system, not only do our organs follow a daily rhythm of heightened activity, but modern research now supports the idea that every cell in the body has its own internal timing mechanism, often referred to as a biological or circadian clock.

5–7 AM: Large Intestine Time

The Large Intestine is most active, preparing the body to eliminate waste from the previous day. This is the best time for a full, natural bowel movement. Drinking warm water upon waking helps stimulate peristalsis and clear toxins. Eating heavy foods now isn't ideal — focus on elimination first.

7–9 AM: Stomach Time

The Stomach's Qi is strong, making this the prime time for a nourishing breakfast. Warm, cooked foods like congee, eggs and steamed or slightly cooked vegetables are ideal. Cold smoothies, raw foods, or skipping breakfast burdens digestion and weakens Spleen Qi.

9–11 AM: Spleen Time

Now the Spleen transforms nutrients into Qi and Blood to fuel the body. Eating a large meal here is discouraged — let the Spleen do its job of distribution. Gentle snacks like fruit (cooked) or bone broth or stewed if digestion is weak may be fine. Energy and focus are naturally strong now.

11 AM–1 PM: Heart Time

The Heart governs circulation and houses the Shen (spirit). Midday is the best time for a balanced lunch that nourishes both body and mind. Include grains, vegetables, and protein to keep Blood moving and support mental clarity. Avoid greasy, heavy meals that can cause sluggishness or palpitations afterward.

1–3 PM: Small Intestine Time

The Small Intestine continues to separate the "clear" (nutrients, fluids) from the "turbid" (waste). This is a good time for light snacks if needed. Overeating here can burden digestion, but a small amount of nuts is fine. This period also supports discernment and decision-making.

3–5 PM: Bladder Time

The Bladder system in TCM helps regulate fluids and eliminate waste. This is a good time for hydration, stretching, or a short walk to support circulation. A small cup of herbal tea is fine, but avoid stimulants like coffee or tea leaf — they overstress the Kidneys.

5–7 PM: Kidney Time

The Kidneys are the foundation of Yin, Yang, and Jing (essence). Energy shifts inward, focusing on conservation and restoration. A light dinner is best — easy-to-digest soups, grains, steamed vegetables, and a small portion of protein. Heavy meals here burden the Kidneys and impair overnight repair.

7–9 PM: Pericardium Time

The Pericardium protects the Heart and governs circulation of Blood, while also buffering the Heart from excessive emotional strain or external stress. This is an ideal time for emotional connection — sharing a meal, conversation, or quiet moments with loved ones. Calming activities such as meditation, journaling, or gentle stretching also nourish Heart energy during this period. Avoid heavy or late-night eating, as it burdens digestion and disrupts circulation. In TCM, the Pericardium is sometimes called the "Heart Protector" or "Minister of the Heart," symbolizing its role as both a physical and emotional shield for your inner center.

9–11 PM: San Jiao (Triple Burner) Time

The San Jiao manages fluid pathways and overall coordination of Qi. This is the best time to be asleep, as the body prepares to shift into deep organ repair. Eating now disrupts the harmonizing function and can create Dampness.

11 PM–1 AM: Gallbladder Time

The Gallbladder governs decision-making and courage in TCM. Deep sleep during this phase allows the body to process fats and restore balance. Staying awake at this time depletes Gallbladder Qi and leads to indecision and poor metabolism.

1–3 AM: Liver Time

The Liver detoxifies, stores Blood, and regulates Qi flow. This is the most important period for deep sleep. Being awake now overstimulates the Liver, leading to irritability, headaches, or red eyes. Heavy late-night meals especially damage this repair cycle.

3–5 AM: Lung Time

The Lungs govern Qi, respiration, and the skin, and this is their key repair period. People with respiratory issues like asthma or chronic cough often wake during these hours because Lung Qi is most active. Waking too early at this time is not ideal, as it can interrupt Lung repair and weaken immunity. If you do wake, gentle breathing can help, but it's best to remain asleep to allow deeper replenishment. This is not a time for eating — instead, the body is preparing for the Large Intestine's elimination phase at 5–7 AM.

Why This Timing Matters

Aligning your daily habits — eating, sleeping, and even pooping — with the body's natural rhythms supports the smooth flow of Qi and helps your organs work more efficiently. When your bathroom habits are irregular, it's worth looking deeper. TCM examines whether the imbalance comes from excess or deficiency, heat or cold, stagnation or dryness — and guides you toward foods, herbs, or lifestyle practices to restore balance. In this way, it's not just about what you do for your health, but when you do it. Living in sync with your internal clock promotes smoother digestion, steadier Qi, and long-term vitality.

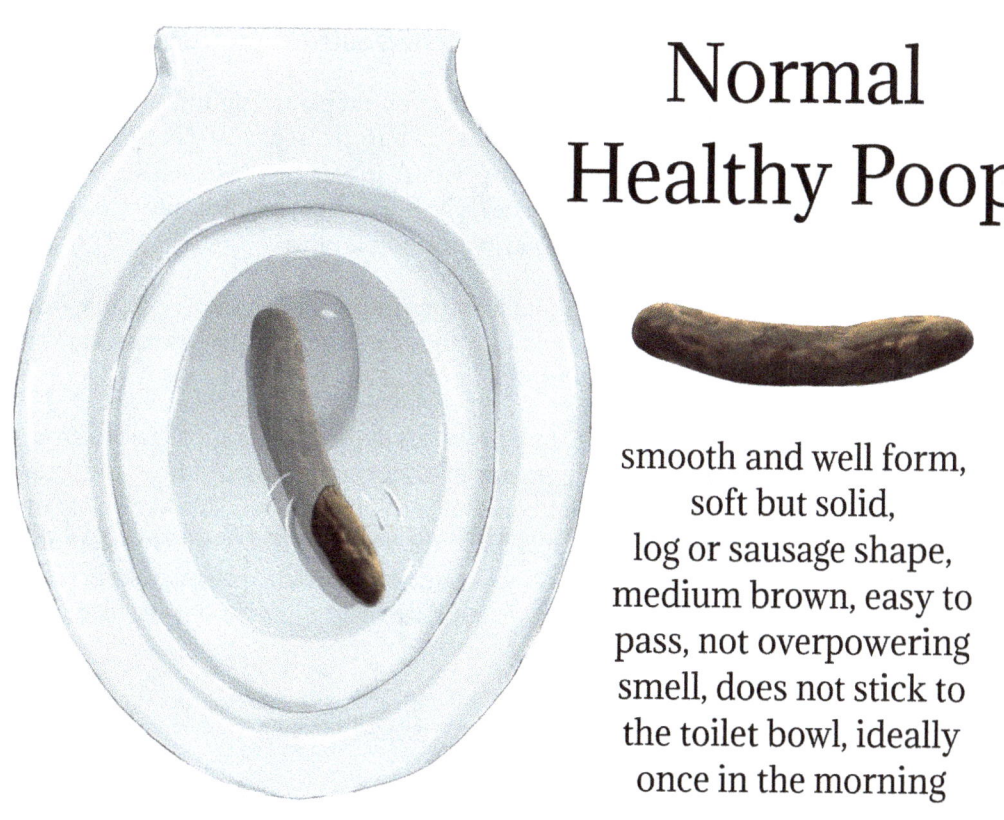

Figure 3.1 Normal healthy poop, banana-shaped, brown or yellow-brown color.

Color. Healthy poop should be brown. This hue is influenced by bile, a fluid produced by the liver that aids in fat digestion. Bile is naturally greenish-yellow, and when it mixes with waste in the small intestine, it gives poop its characteristic brown color.

Consistency. Poop should be firm with a smooth surface and maintain this shape in water. When poop is firm with a smooth surface, it is easy to pass without being too sticky or watery.

Shape. The ideal poop should have a cylindrical shape, resembling a banana, sausage, or snake. This reflects a healthy large intestine without any obstructions, polyps, fissures, or twists.

Frequency. As discussed earlier, one bowel movement per day is generally considered a sign of a healthy digestive system. In TCM, a daily bowel movement soon after waking in the morning is ideal.

Texture. The surface of your poop should appear smooth and uniform. It should not be fluffy, lumpy or cracked.

Weight. The amount of daily poop is around 100-200 grams (3.5 - 7 oz). However, this can vary depending on your diet. If you're eating a lot but not producing much waste, it could indicate a blockage.

Buoyancy. Healthy poop should sink in water. This suggests efficient digestion with full nutrient extraction and absorption. The remaining waste is compacted into dense poop that sinks. Floating stool may indicate poor digestion, as it suggests that undigested food is present.

Lack of Undigested Food. Normal stool in TCM should not contain undigested food particles. The Spleen and Stomach, which are key digestive organs in TCM, should effectively process and transform food.

Ease of Passing. Normal stool should be easy to pass without straining or discomfort. Difficulty in passing stool can indicate imbalances in the digestive system, such as excess internal heat, lack of fluid or Blood and Qi deficiency leading to constipation.

Odor. While poop does have an odor, extremely foul or unusual odors can be a sign of digestive issues or imbalances.

Several factors can influence the appearance of your poop. What you eat plays a significant role in determining the color, consistency, and smell of your poop. For instance, a diet rich in red meat can lead to darker-colored stool. Certain medications can also affect the appearance of your poop. Antibiotics, for instance, can cause loose stools. If you have digestive problems like constipation or diarrhea, they can alter the appearance of your poop. Lastly, infections, such as a stomach bug, can also impact the way your poop looks.

Understanding these TCM principles of poop frequency and appearance can offer valuable insights into your overall health. By paying attention to your bathroom habits and making necessary adjustments to your diet and lifestyle, you can strive for optimal digestive health and well-being.

Additionally, it's important to note that TCM diagnosis is holistic, taking into account various aspects of a person's health, lifestyle, and individual constitution. The frequency of abnormal stools and how consistently they occur are important factors in TCM assessment. If abnormal stools happen only occasionally like once a month, it may be less of a concern compared to more frequent occurrences like once a week, which could indicate an imbalance that needs attention. If you have concerns about your digestive health or experience changes in bowel habits, consult with a medical practitioner who can help determine an appropriate course of action to restore the balance.

Understanding the Different types of Stool Odors

Have you ever noticed that your stool smells different from time to time?

The smell of your stool can provide information regarding the type of food consumed and how well it is being digested. Here are some common stool odors and what they may indicate:

Foul Odor. Foul-smelling feces can be related to the consumption of excessive protein and lipids. When you eat more protein and fat than your body can efficiently digest, it can lead to the production of odorous compounds during the digestive process.

Sour Odor. A sour smell in feces might result from the overconsumption of carbohydrates. When carbohydrates ferment in the colon due to the action of gut bacteria, gasses, and compounds are produced, contributing to sour odors.

Fishy Odor. A fishy smell in feces could be linked to the consumption of an excess of raw, cold, or iced drinks and foods. Cold or raw foods and drinks can sometimes disrupt the digestive process, leading to unusual odors.

Rotten Odor. A rotten smell in feces may indeed be associated with food poisoning or food retention. When the body struggles to digest or eliminate certain foods, it can result in the production of rotten-smelling compounds. Food poisoning is a common cause of this issue.

Normal Smell. Ideally, stool should have a mild, earthy odor without being foul or overly pungent. It's considered normal for stool to have some odor, as this is a natural byproduct of the digestive process and the action of gut bacteria. The smell should not be overpowering or offensive.

Monitoring changes in stool odor, along with other digestive symptoms, can be beneficial for assessing your digestive health. If you notice persistent or concerning changes in stool odor, it's advisable to consult a healthcare professional to determine the underlying cause and receive appropriate guidance or treatment.

In the following chapters, we'll explore different types of color, abnormal stools, what they can tell you about your health, and how you can make lifestyle adjustments. We will also present Traditional Chinese Medicine practices to address these issues.

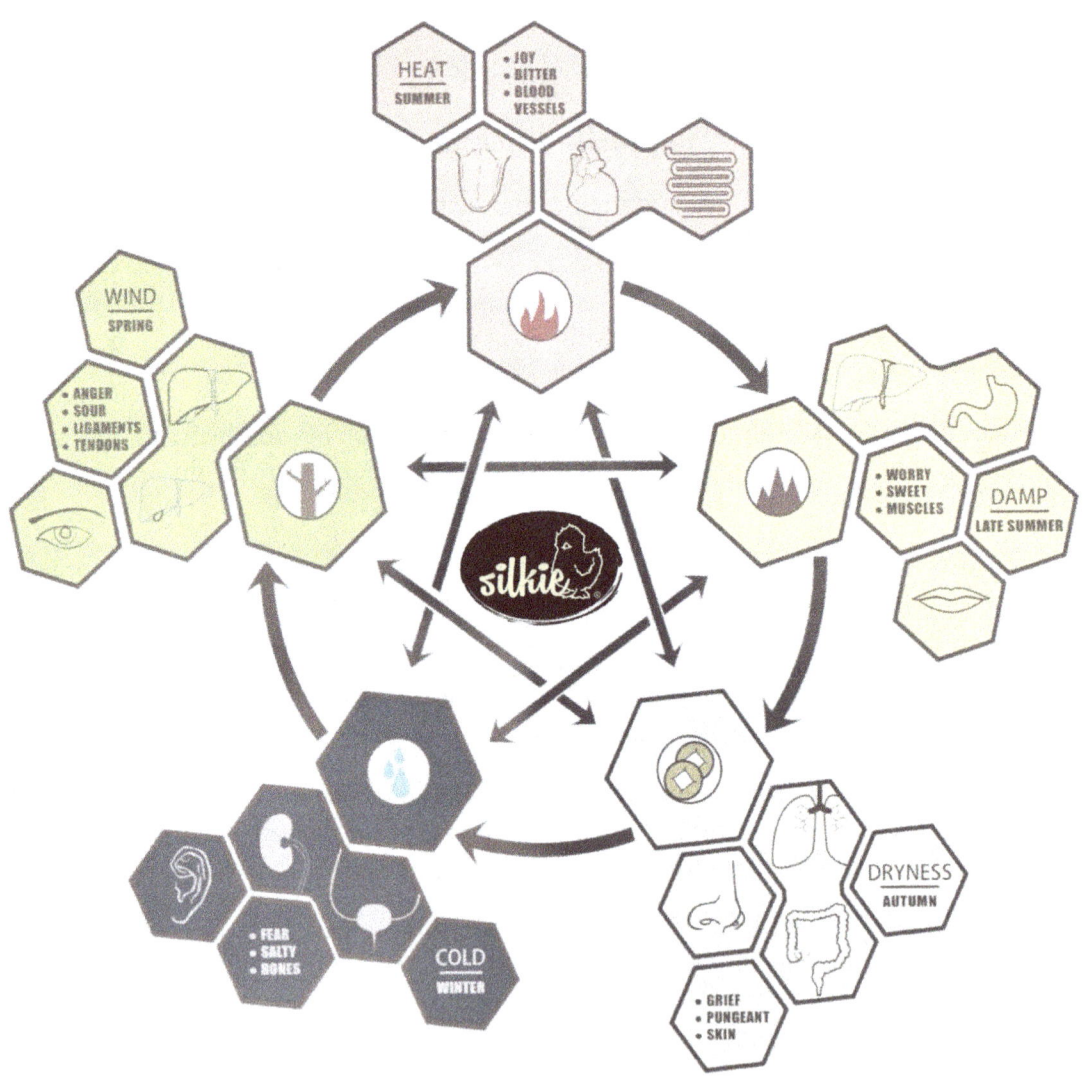

Understanding the Different Colors of Stools

Have you ever noticed your poop isn't brown?

We don't often think about the color of our poop — but it's one of the most reliable daily indicators of how your digestive system and internal organs are functioning. In TCM, stool color offers a window into the harmony of your body's internal landscape. Each color reflects how well your Qi (energy), Blood, Yin, and Yang are balanced, as well as how smoothly your organs — especially the Spleen, Liver, and Stomach — are performing their roles.

Before we jump into what color changes might mean, it's important to note that not all shifts in stool color are signs of illness. Sometimes, what you see in the toilet is simply the result of what you've eaten or what your body is processing that day.

When Food Causes Temporary Color Changes

Certain foods contain strong natural pigments or additives that can temporarily alter the color of your stool. These changes are usually harmless and disappear once the food passes through your system.

Green stool is often caused by eating large amounts of leafy greens like spinach, kale, or wheatgrass. In some cases, rapid transit through the intestines (when food moves too quickly) can also leave the stool green, as bile pigments haven't had time to break down. Artificial coloring in candies, drinks, or supplements can also be responsible.

Red stool may appear after eating beets, red dragon fruit, red gelatin, or brightly dyed foods. While red can sometimes indicate bleeding in the lower digestive tract, if the color disappears within a day and there are no other symptoms, food is the most likely cause.

Yellow or orange stool can occur after consuming foods high in beta-carotene, such as carrots, pumpkin, and sweet potatoes, or from turmeric. In these cases, the stool is typically soft and well-formed, with no signs of illness.

Dark brown or black stool may result from iron-rich foods (like red meat or liver), iron supplements, activated charcoal, or black licorice. These sources darken stool naturally and should not be mistaken for bleeding if the person feels well.

If the color change is brief and clearly related to diet, it's usually nothing to worry about. But if unusual colors — especially black, pale, or bright red — persist and can't be traced back to food, it's worth investigating. In TCM, such color changes may reflect deeper imbalances in the Spleen, Liver, or digestive Qi, rather than being caused by bacteria alone.

In this chapter, we'll explore different stool colors and their significance. Some stool colors might even be a medical red flag. Let's break it down:

1. Brown Stool. It's a common color for most people, but Not Always the "Perfect" Shape. While medium brown stool is often seen as a sign of good digestive health, it doesn't automatically mean the shape or texture is healthy. You can have brown-colored poop that's still too dry, too loose, cracked, or oddly shaped — signs that something may be off with your digestion, even if the color looks "normal." So while brown is a good baseline, we need to consider the full picture: shape, texture, frequency, and ease of passage.

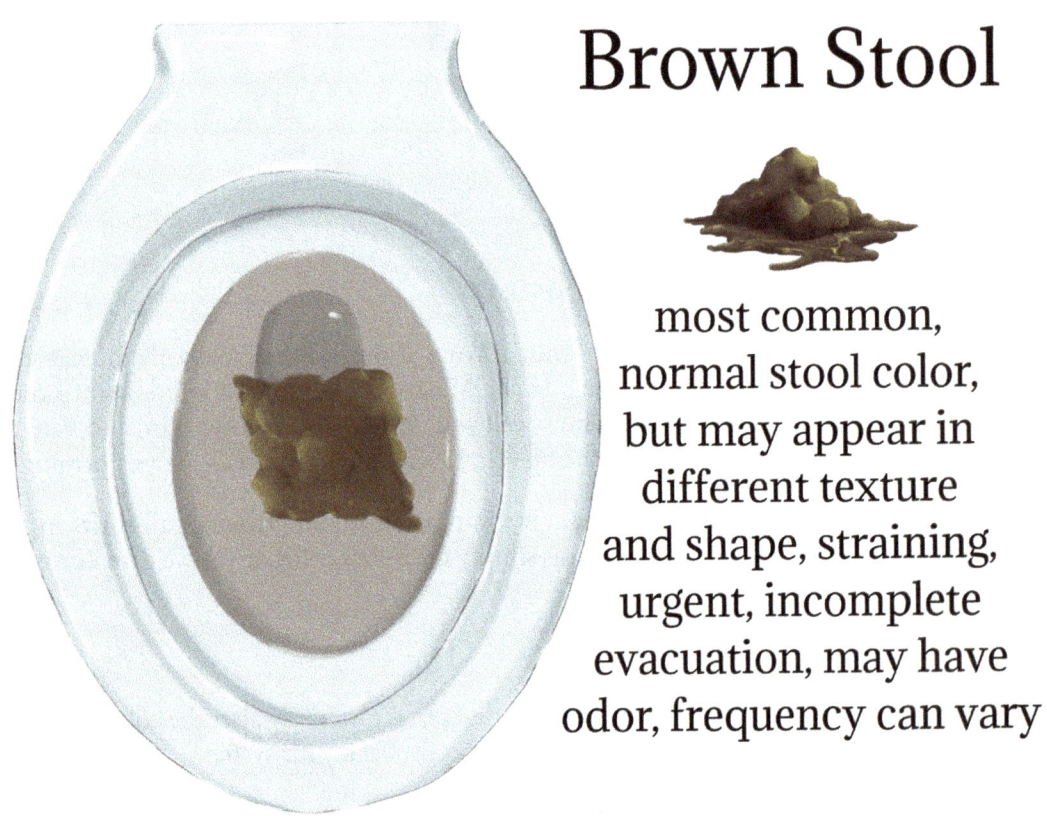

Brown Stool

most common, normal stool color, but may appear in different texture and shape, straining, urgent, incomplete evacuation, may have odor, frequency can vary

Figure 5.1 Brown stool, Spleen and Stomach Qi are functioning properly.

The brown color itself comes mainly from bile — a digestive fluid produced by the Liver. When fresh, bile is yellowish, but after spending time stored in the Gallbladder, it turns green. Once food enters the Small Intestine, bile is released into the duodenum to help break down fats. Most of this bile is reabsorbed at the end of the Small Intestine and recycled back to the Liver. Only about 10% continues into the Large Intestine, where it mixes with undigested food. This final blend, combined with the action of gut bacteria, gives stool its typical chocolate brown or yellow-brown hue.

It's important to remember that even though brown stool is considered "normal," it doesn't automatically mean everything is in balance. Temporary changes in stool color may happen with dietary shifts or minor digestive fluctuations, but persistent issues — like very dark, pale, or oddly shaped stool — can signal deeper imbalances. In Traditional Chinese Medicine, these might reflect issues with the Liver, Gallbladder, or Spleen systems. If you experience ongoing digestive changes, it's wise to consult both a medical professional and a TCM practitioner to assess what's going on beneath the surface and help guide your body back to balance.

2. Dark Yellow Stool. Darker yellow stool can sometimes be a normal variation depending on diet — especially if you've eaten foods rich in yellow pigments like carrots, sweet potatoes, or turmeric. However, if the color is noticeably darker than usual and persistent, it can be an abnormal sign and may be related to bilirubin. Bilirubin is a yellow compound produced during the breakdown of red blood cells and is normally processed by the Liver and excreted in the bile, which gives stool its brown color. In Western medicine, darker yellow stool can also be seen in people with faster intestinal transit time (like mild diarrhea), or early stages of malabsorption, where bile hasn't fully oxidized to the usual brown.

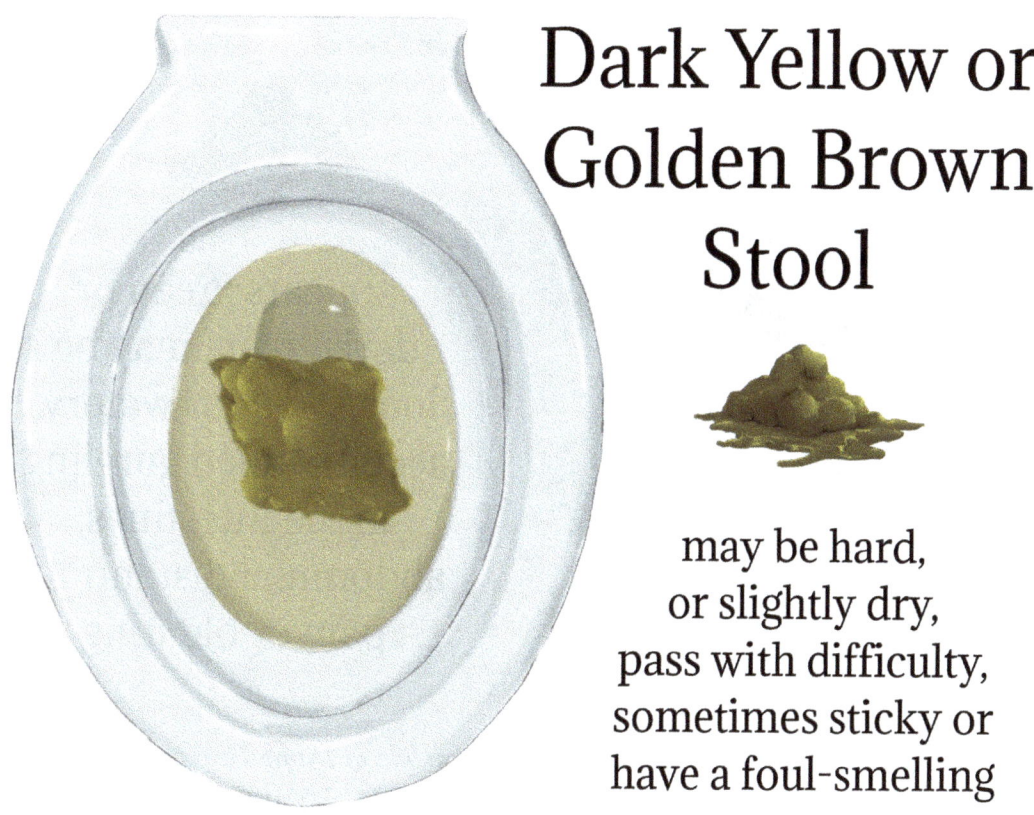

Dark Yellow or Golden Brown Stool

may be hard, or slightly dry, pass with difficulty, sometimes sticky or have a foul-smelling

Figure 5.2 Dark yellow stool, Damp-Heat in Liver and Gallbladder.

In Traditional Chinese Medicine, dark yellow stool is often seen as a sign of Damp-Heat in the Liver and Gallbladder. This pattern arises when internal Heat (from spicy, greasy, or fried foods, stress, or external pathogens) combines with Dampness (fluid stagnation from improper digestion or Spleen Qi deficiency). The result is foul-smelling, sticky, or loose stool that appears dark yellow or golden. You may also notice symptoms like abdominal discomfort, bloating, bad breath, thirst with little desire to drink, or a yellow, greasy coating on the tongue.

TCM treatment focuses on clearing Heat and resolving Dampness, often with herbal formulas and dietary changes — favoring light, cooling, and easy-to-digest foods while avoiding rich, oily, or spicy meals. If the color persists, especially with digestive discomfort or fatigue, it's wise to consult both a TCM practitioner and a medical provider to rule out liver, gallbladder, or intestinal issues.

3. Green Stool. Eating a lot of green, leafy vegetables like spinach or kale or foods with green food coloring can cause stools to be green. Some iron supplements can also cause poop to be green. If the cause isn't food or supplement intake, then dark green stool, especially if it's accompanied by a rancid smell can signal a liver or intestine problem.

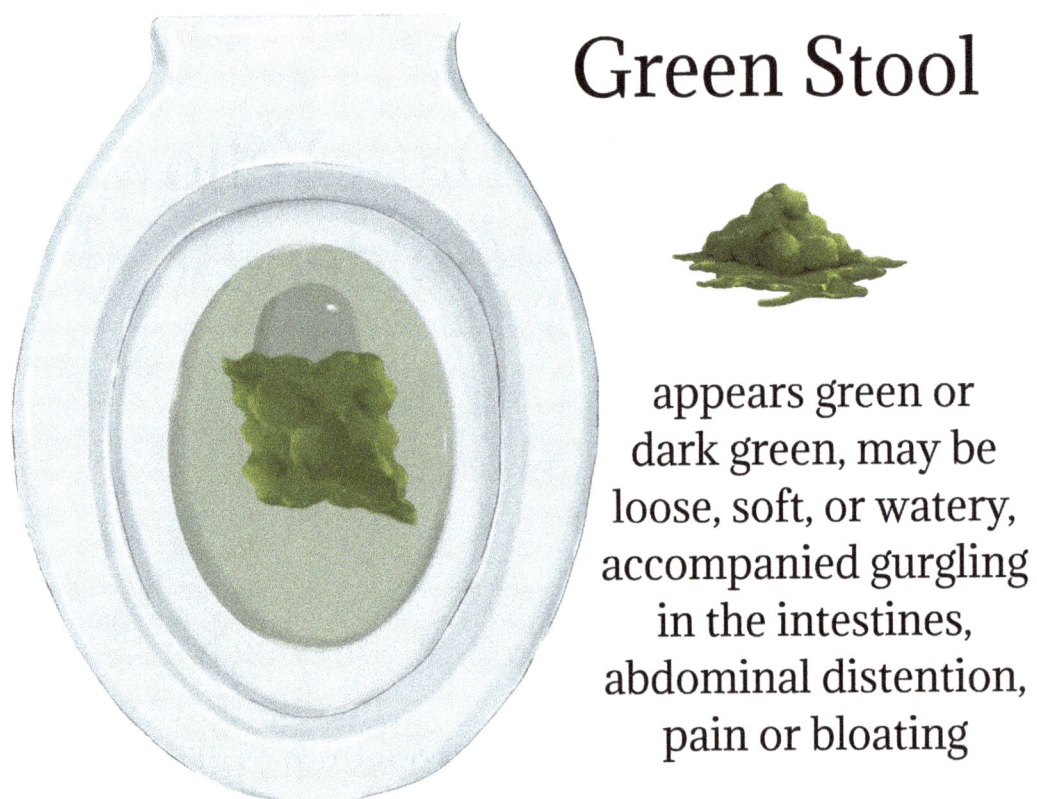

Green Stool

appears green or dark green, may be loose, soft, or watery, accompanied gurgling in the intestines, abdominal distention, pain or bloating

Figure 5.3 Green Stool, Liver Qi Stagnation, too much bile, or Damp-Heat in the Intestines, Spleen and Stomach Deficiency with Coldness.

The TCM pattern of Liver Qi stagnation is a common imbalance often caused by emotional stress, frustration, or anger. When green stool appears alongside emotional tension, it frequently points to this pattern. Another possible explanation for green stool is Damp Heat in the Intestines. In general, the greener the stool, the higher the concentration of bile, the digestive fluid produced by the liver and stored in the gallbladder to help break down fats. Green stools can indicate an issue in the small intestine where less bile is reabsorbed and more flows into the large intestine.

If green stool is accompanied by diarrhea and pain in the lower right abdomen, more serious conditions such as intestinal inflammation or tumors could be involved. However, the most common cause is acute gastroenteritis. In such cases, inflammation in the small intestine impairs its ability to reabsorb bile, resulting in stool that appears dark green or even blackish-green. This pattern reflects how infection or inflammation in the intestines can disrupt the digestive process and influence stool color.

4. Light Yellow Stool. In Western medicine, light yellow stool can be an indicator that bile is not reaching the intestines properly. Bile, produced by the Liver and stored in the Gallbladder, is what gives stool its normal brown color. If bile flow is reduced — due to issues like liver disease, gallstones, bile duct blockage, or even pancreas problems — stool can appear pale, clay-colored, or light yellow. It may also float, smell foul, or look greasy if fat digestion is compromised.

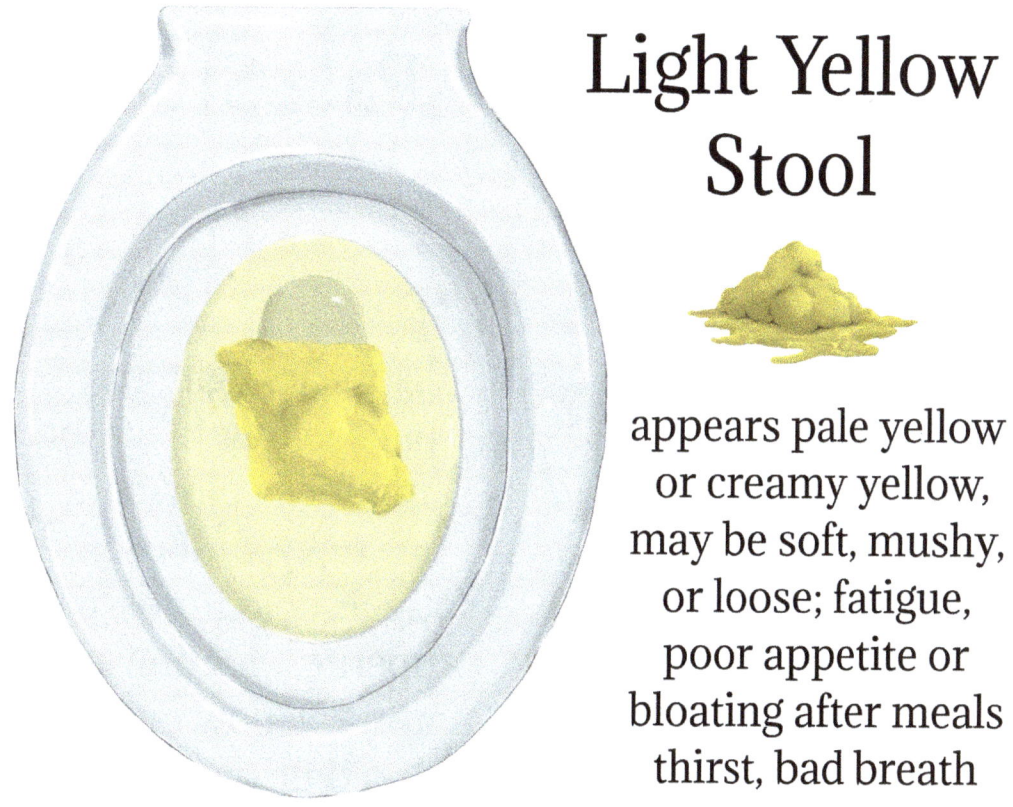

Figure 5.4 Light yellow stool, weak Spleen Qi Deficiency with Dampness.

In Traditional Chinese Medicine, light yellow stool is most often linked to Spleen Qi Deficiency or the presence of Dampness. The Spleen in TCM is not only the anatomical spleen but also a functional system that includes aspects of the pancreas. Its primary role is to transform food into Qi and Blood and to distribute fluids throughout the body. When the Spleen is weakened — often by overconsumption of cold, raw, greasy, or difficult-to-digest foods, as well as by emotional strain or chronic overthinking — its transformative power is diminished.

As a result, food and fluids are not fully cooked or processed. Instead, they linger in the digestive tract in a semi-digested form, which can create stools that are light in color, mushy, or greasy. This indicates a lack of digestive fire rather than excess Heat. From a TCM perspective, this reflects a weakened Spleen Qi, sometimes tipping toward Spleen Yang Deficiency, where there is not enough warmth or energy to properly transform food.

Addressing light yellow stool involves strengthening digestion. From a TCM view, this may include warm, cooked foods, avoiding cold/raw meals, and using herbal formulas to tonify the Spleen and drain Dampness. However, if this type of stool persists or worsens, a medical check-up is essential to rule out liver or bile-related issues.

5. Pale, Gray, or Clay-Colored Stool. Typically indicates a bile insufficiency problem. When bile production is insufficient or when the passage of bile to the small intestine is blocked, the stool lacks its normal brown color and becomes unusually light. This can be a serious medical concern. If pale stool is accompanied by yellowing of the eyes or skin and dark, tea-colored urine, it may signal obstructive jaundice — a condition most commonly caused by pancreatic cancer, bile duct cancer, or, less frequently, a gallstone blocking the common bile duct. Prompt medical evaluation is strongly recommended.

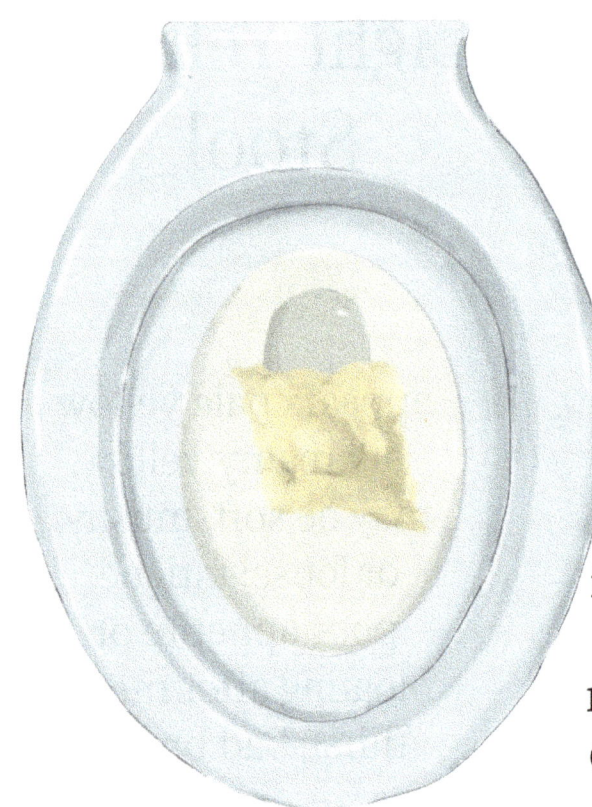

Pale Stool

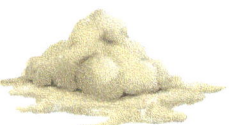

appears light gray, pale yellow, beige, or whitish color, soft, sticky, or loose, fatigue, cold limbs, poor appetite, bloating, mild nausea, yellow eyes, tea-colored urine, itchy skin

Figure 5.5 Pale stool, Liver Qi Stagnation, Gallbladder Dampness, or Spleen Yang deficiency.

In Traditional Chinese Medicine, pale or grayish-white stool may reflect one of three possible internal imbalances: Liver Qi stagnation, Gallbladder dysfunction, dampness obstructing the bile ducts, or Spleen Yang deficiency. The correct pattern is identified by accompanying symptoms. Emotional stress and abdominal distention point to Liver Qi stagnation. Nausea and a bitter taste suggest Gallbladder Dampness. A cold sensation in the abdomen, chronic fatigue, and digestive weakness are signs of Spleen Yang deficiency. Each of these patterns is treated strategically with herbs or acupuncture points along with dietary and lifestyle modifications aimed at restoring proper bile production and flow, supporting digestion, and rebalancing the affected organ system.

6. Red or Dark Red Stool. Sometimes, red stool is simply the result of eating red-colored foods like beets, red dragon fruit, or foods containing artificial red dyes. In these cases, there is no actual bleeding — just a temporary change in color. However, when bright red blood appears on, around or mixed in the stool, especially if it's visible on toilet paper or in the water, it may indicate bleeding in the lower part of the digestive tract. Common causes include hemorrhoids, anal fissures, inflammatory bowel disease, or colorectal polyps.

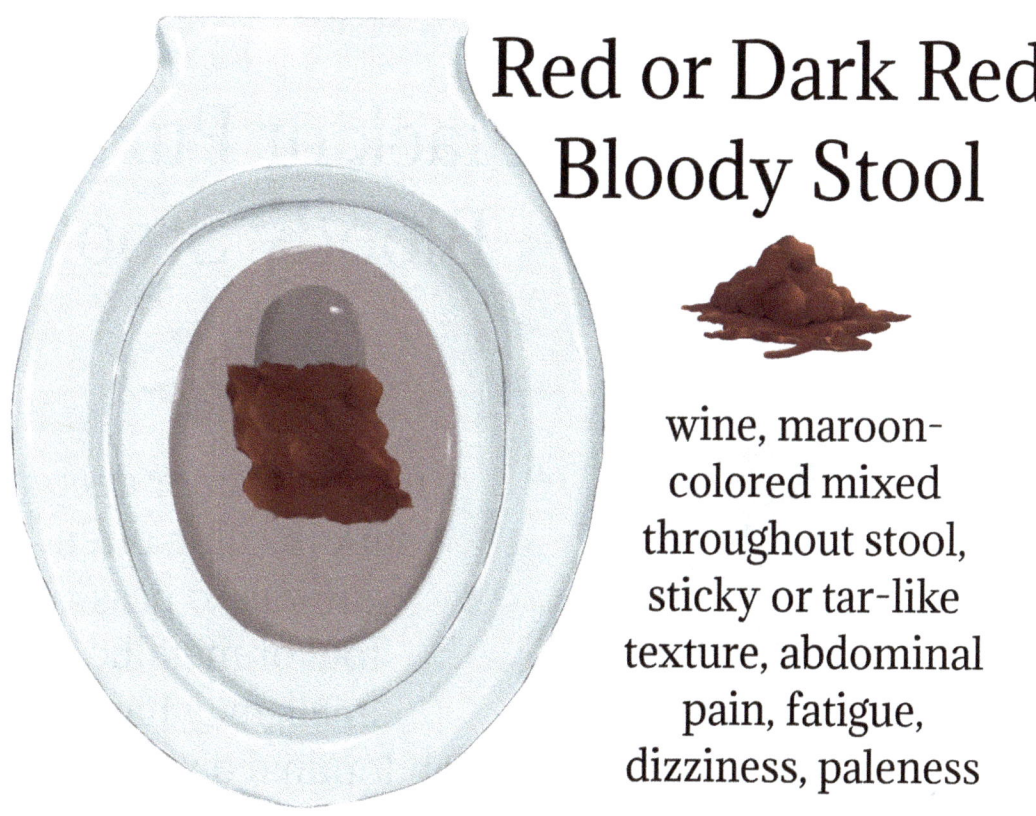

Figure 5.6 Red or dark red stool, Blood Heat, and Intestinal imbalance, usually from lower digestive tract bleeding.

From a Traditional Chinese Medicine perspective, this often points to a pattern known as Blood Heat. Blood Heat causes the blood to move more recklessly, increasing the likelihood of it leaking out of the vessels. This condition is often triggered by a diet rich in hot and spicy foods, emotional stress that disrupts Liver and Intestinal balance, or prolonged constipation that leads to straining. In other cases, if someone is already Qi-deficient — especially in the Spleen — the body may not be able to hold the Blood in the vessels, leading to bleeding even without excess Heat. TCM treatment would focus on clearing Heat, cooling the Blood, and tonifying the Spleen to better contain the Blood and prevent recurrence. If blood is visible, prompt medical attention is advised.

7. Black Stool. Black stool can be alarming, especially when it appears tar-like, sticky, and has a foul odor. In Western medicine, this often points to bleeding in the upper digestive tract, such as the stomach or the first part of the small intestine. When blood travels a longer distance through the intestines before being excreted, it gets broken down by digestive enzymes, turning it dark brown or black. This condition is known as melena and may be a sign of serious issues like stomach ulcers, gastritis, or even tumors. Certain foods like black licorice, blueberries and iron supplements can also cause stool to turn black, but they usually don't cause the sticky, tar-like texture associated with bleeding.

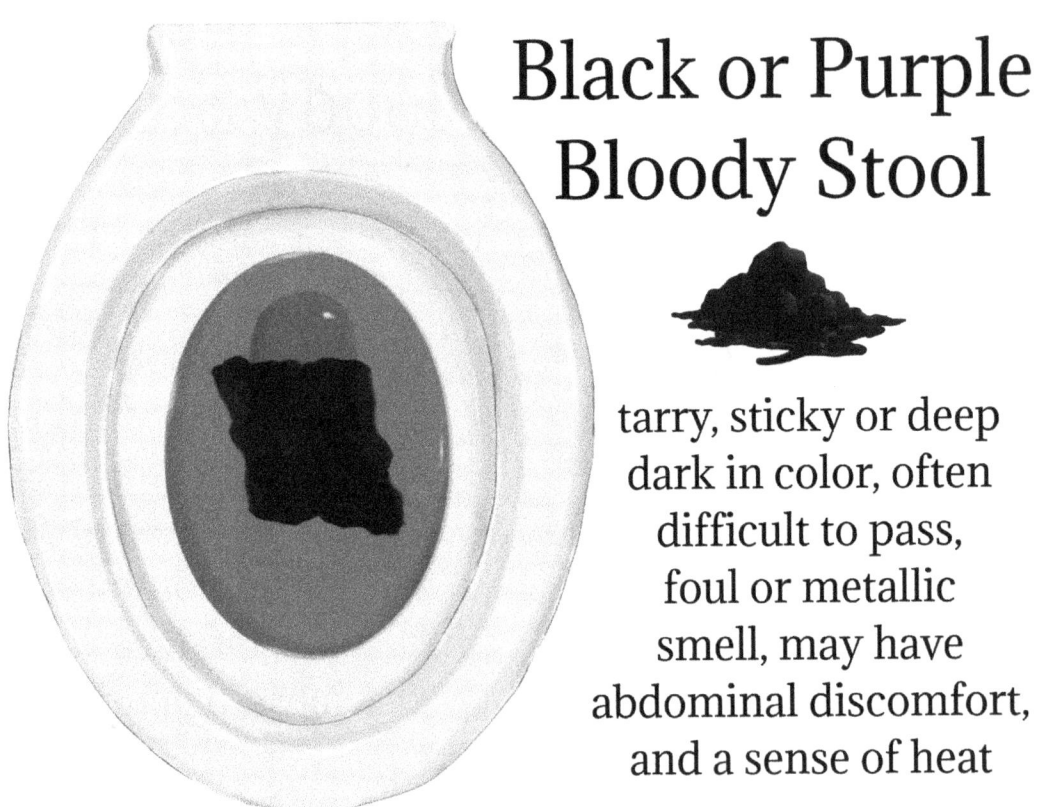

Figure 5.7 Black stool, Spleen Qi Deficiency, Liver Qi Stagnation, Blood Stasis, or chronic Heat in the Stomach or Intestines, usually from upper digestive tract.

In Traditional Chinese Medicine, black stool is often seen as a sign of Blood Stasis or Stagnant Blood, especially when the stool is dark, thick, and accompanied by pain or a sensation of fullness. This condition typically arises from long-standing Heat in the Stomach or Intestines, which "agitates" the Blood, causing it to move recklessly and escape the vessels. Over time, this unregulated movement can result in internal bleeding. The longer the blood remains in the body before being eliminated, the darker it becomes — hence the black appearance. Black stool may also suggest Spleen Qi Deficiency failing to contain Blood in the vessels, or a Yin Deficiency with Empty Heat, where internal dryness causes blood vessels to become fragile. Emotionally, chronic stress, frustration, or anger can stagnate Liver Qi, which then transforms into Heat and invades the Stomach, increasing the likelihood of bleeding.

While TCM can offer long-term support — such as cooling the Blood, nourishing Yin, and strengthening the Spleen — black stool is considered a serious warning sign in both medical systems. Immediate evaluation by a healthcare provider is crucial to rule out life-threatening conditions and determine the appropriate course of action.

8. Fresh Red, Bloody Stool. In more serious cases, fresh red blood in the stool or vomit may be a sign of internal bleeding due to advanced liver disease, such as cirrhosis. When the liver becomes scarred and hardened, it increases pressure in the portal vein system, leading to the formation of fragile, swollen blood vessels — called varices — in the esophagus or stomach. If these varices rupture, they can cause large amounts of bleeding. Blood may be vomited or passed through the anus, appearing as fresh red blood if the bleeding is rapid and near the exit.

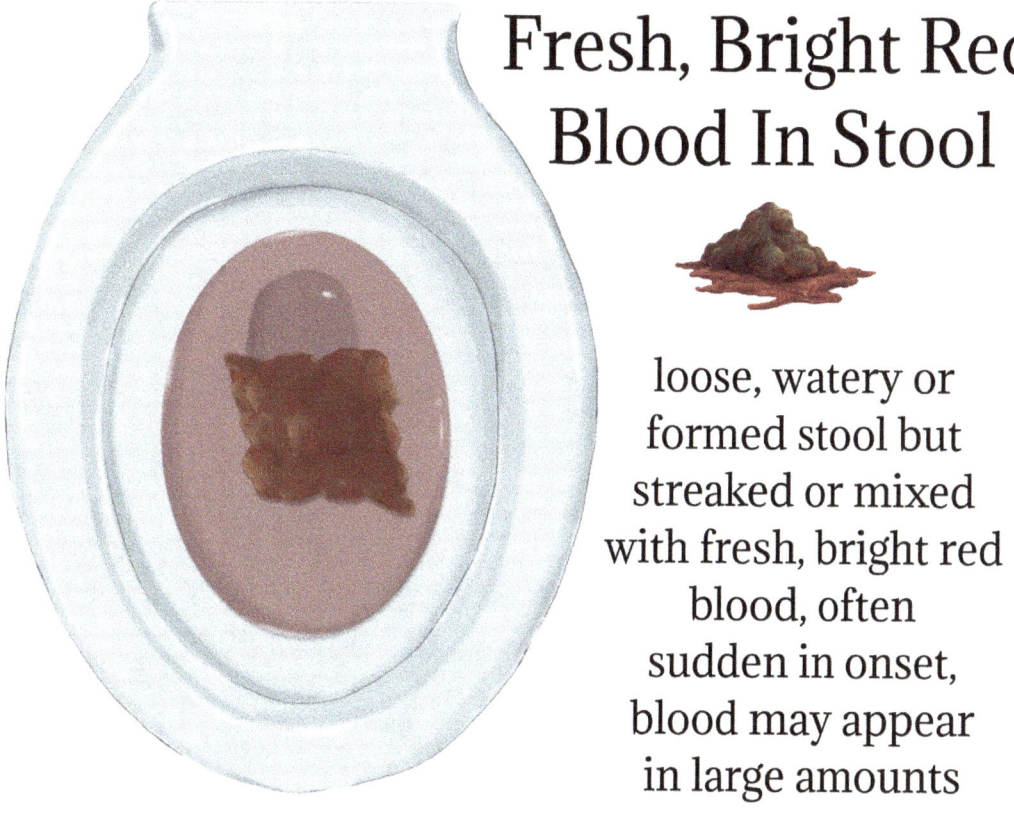

Figure 5.8 Fresh, bright red, bloody stool, Chronic Liver Qi Stagnation, Damp-Heat accumulation, and Blood Stasis damaging the Liver collaterals, gradually leading to vessel fragility and bleeding, usually from cirrhosis or variceal bleeding.

This is considered a medical emergency and requires immediate hospital care. In Traditional Chinese Medicine, this kind of bleeding is often associated with Liver Blood Stasis or Liver Fire, which disturbs the normal flow of Qi and Blood and causes the blood vessels to become fragile. It may also reflect an underlying Yin Deficiency, where internal dryness weakens vessel integrity, or Spleen Qi Deficiency, which fails to hold blood in the vessels. While emergency care must come first, long-term TCM strategies may be used to harmonize the Liver, strengthen the Spleen, and cool or nourish the Blood to prevent recurrence and support recovery.

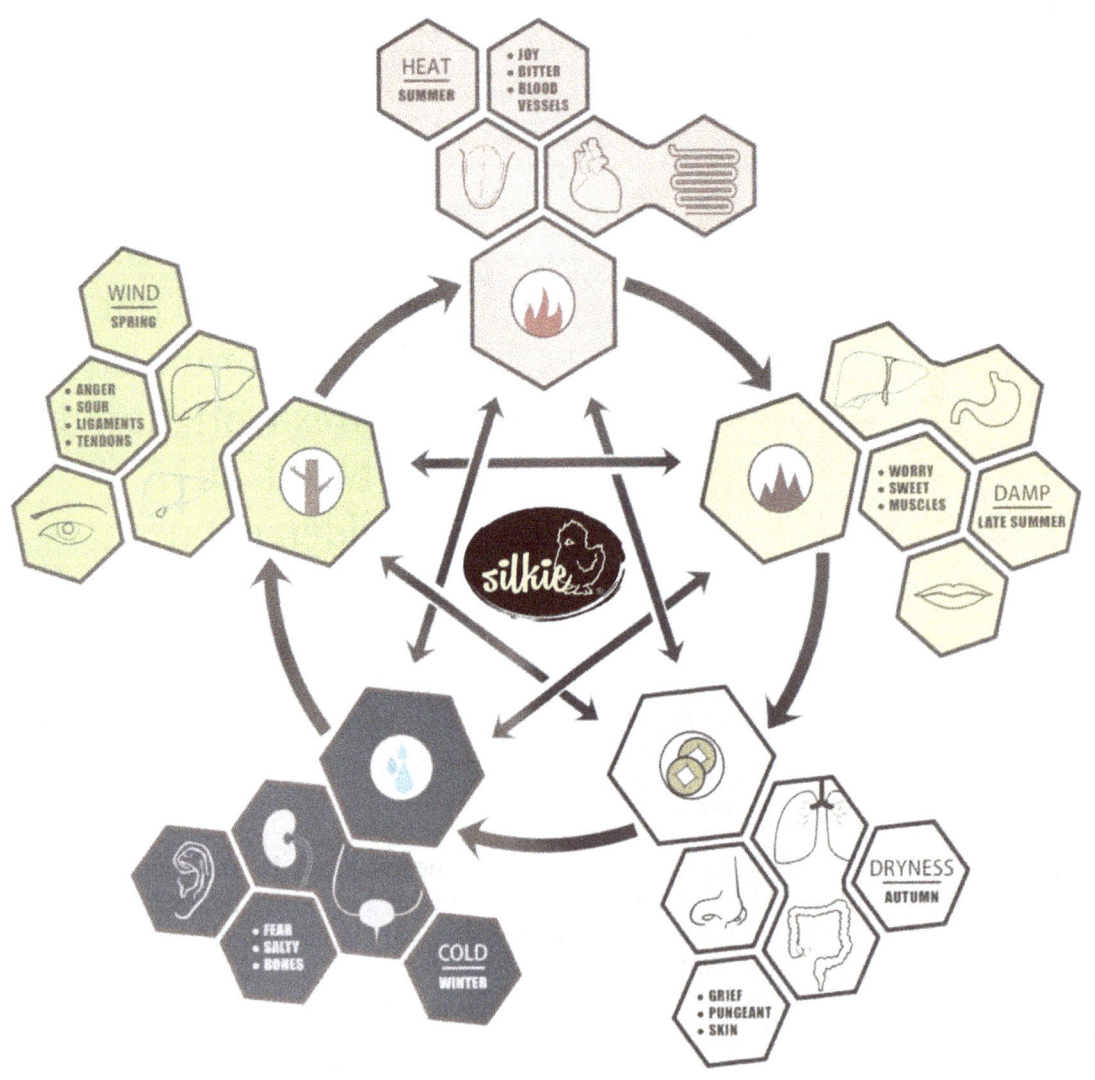

Understanding Stool Types
Bumpy, Lumpy Stool

Have you ever wondered why your stool has different shapes and textures?

In both TCM and modern health perspectives, your poop offers important clues about how well your digestive system is functioning and whether your body is absorbing nutrients properly. Now let's discuss the common stool types based on shape, texture, and frequency - if you pay close attention, it can reveal a lot.

1. Bumpy or Lumpy Stool - Sign of Kidney Deficiency

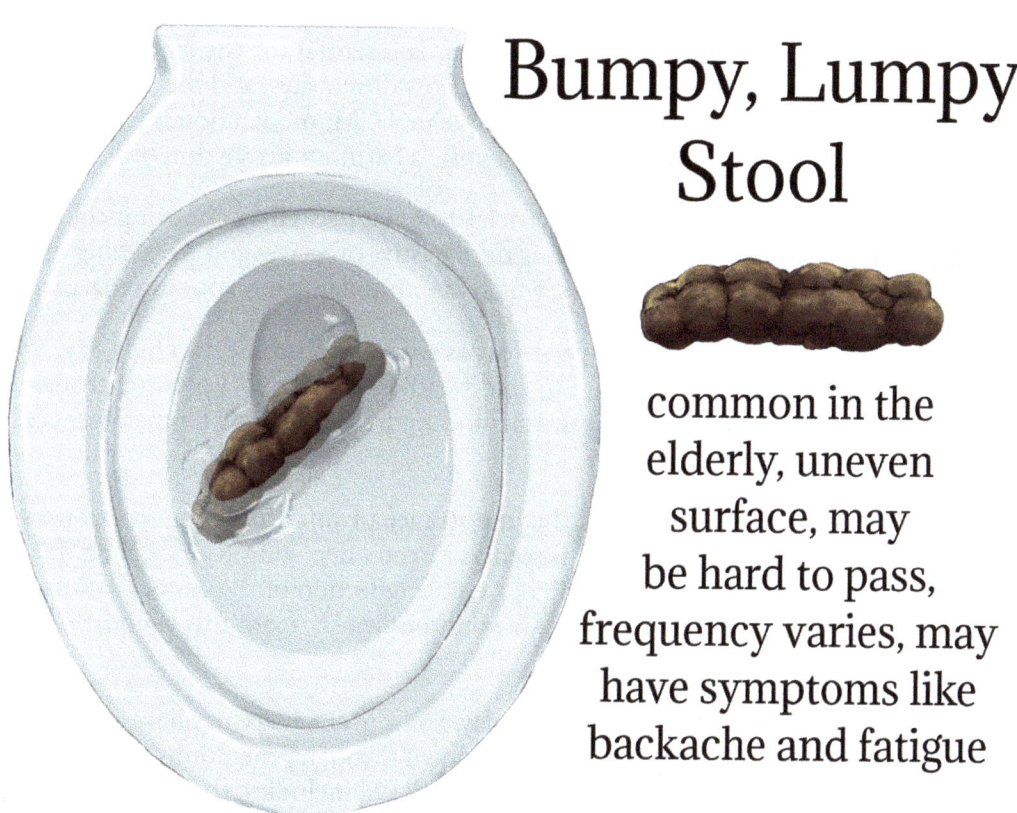

Bumpy, Lumpy Stool

common in the elderly, uneven surface, may be hard to pass, frequency varies, may have symptoms like backache and fatigue

Figure 6.1 Bumpy or lumpy stool, Kidney Deficiency or long-term Qi and Fluid Deficiency.

What it Means: Bumpy or lumpy stool, characterized by an uneven surface, indicates Kidney Deficiency. The Kidneys are the foundation of Yin and Yang in the body and are closely tied to the body's fluid metabolism. When Kidney Yin is deficient, there's a lack of moisture to soften and lubricate the stool. When Kidney Yang is weak, there's not enough warmth and movement to propel the waste smoothly. Both conditions can lead to dry, uneven, or segmented stools that are hard to pass. This condition is more common in the elderly, but common does not mean healthy. Unlike hard, dry, compacted stools which occur once a day or once every few days and can be difficult to pass, bumpy stools are more moist and vary in frequency from once every couple of days to multiple bowel movements per day. Additionally, bumpy stools can be easy or difficult to pass.

Underlying Causes

The Kidneys in Traditional Chinese Medicine are not just filters. The Kidneys are the very wellspring of our vitality, the deep roots from which all our energy and essence flow. Think of their inherent energy, Yuan Qi or Source Qi, like a finite inheritance we're born with. As we journey through life, this precious reserve naturally ebbs, particularly as we age – it's the gentle, inevitable rhythm of time, like the slow fading of twilight. This natural decline makes our elders more susceptible to what we call Kidney deficiency.

But it's not just the ticking clock that can strain these vital organs. Our modern lives, often a whirlwind of emotional, mental, and physical demands, can rapidly deplete this precious Kidney Qi if we don't prioritize rest and rejuvenation. Think of prolonged stress as a relentless storm, constantly battering our reserves, much like how chronic stress can weaken the adrenal glands in Western medicine. This constant "fight or flight" mode burns through our energy stores, leaving the Kidneys weary. Even the nature of our work can take its toll. The intense focus required for writing or consulting can create a mental strain that, when severe, keeps the mind racing into the night, stealing precious sleep and further draining Kidney energy. Similarly, professions demanding heavy physical labor relentlessly tax the body, and without adequate recovery, this overexertion chips away at the Kidney's Yang energy, the warming and active force within.

Interestingly, the opposite of this relentless activity — a sedentary lifestyle — can also contribute to Kidney deficiency. Movement, like a gentle breeze through a garden, is essential for the smooth circulation of vital energy throughout the body. When we become stagnant, this flow diminishes, and the Kidneys don't receive the stimulation they need to thrive. This highlights a core principle in TCM: moderation is key. Just as nature needs the balance of sun and rain for life to flourish, our bodies require a harmonious rhythm of activity and rest.

Even something as fundamental as our diet plays a crucial role. Consistently choosing cold, raw, or heavily processed foods is like dousing our internal fire, hindering the digestive processes and weakening the warming Yang energy of the Kidneys. The same goes for icy beverages, which can put a damper on our internal metabolic furnace.

Our external environment also has a profound impact. Just as we seek warmth on a chilly day, our Kidneys are sensitive to cold and dampness. Prolonged exposure to cold weather or living in a persistently damp climate can directly deplete Kidney Yang. Even in warmer regions, a significant drop in evening temperatures can expose us to environmental cold, subtly draining our reserves.

In the realm of personal habits, TCM emphasizes the importance of mindful living. Excessive sexual activity, viewed as a significant expenditure of vital essence, is seen as directly depleting Kidney Yang. It's even said that in men, the telltale sign can appear as a receding hairline, a visible reflection of the Kidney's diminished strength. Engaging in overly frequent sexual activity is seen as drawing too heavily from this foundational wellspring of energy.

Beyond these lifestyle factors, there are other influences at play. Some individuals may have a constitutional predisposition to Kidney Deficiency, an inherited tendency passed down through generations. Furthermore, prolonged or recurring illnesses act as a persistent drain on the body's overall Qi, including that of the Kidneys. Finally, the often-underestimated importance of rest and sleep cannot be overstated. Inadequate and disrupted sleep patterns place a significant strain on the Kidney system, hindering its ability to replenish and contributing to deficiency.

While we can't rewrite our genetic code, we absolutely have the power to influence its expression through our lifestyle choices. While TCM offers powerful tools to aid recovery from illness and build resilience, prioritizing rest and sleep is perhaps where we hold the most immediate control. Ignoring persistent insomnia is like leaving a tap running on our precious Kidney reserves, insidiously depleting them and potentially leading to a cascade of more serious health issues down the line. Seeking professional help for sleep disturbances is therefore a crucial step in safeguarding the very root of our vitality.

Why The Kidneys Are Important To Our Body

In Traditional Chinese Medicine, the Kidneys are super important because they are the headquarters for the body's energy and vitality. The Kidneys impact on health goes far beyond the physiological role of filtering blood. The Kidneys are viewed as the foundation of life and play a central role in how well we age. The robustness of the Kidneys is closely tied to longevity. When the Kidneys are strong, the body has more energy, resilience, and vitality, which helps slow the visible and internal signs of aging.

Like a battery storing energy, the Kidneys store a vital essence called, *"Jing"*, which naturally declines over time – but can be preserved through healthy lifestyle practices and herbal support. Jing is the most fundamental substance for growth, development, fertility, and vitality. There are two types of essence: Prenatal Jing (inherited from your parents) and Postnatal Jing (produced from food and air). The Kidneys store both, and Jing depletion is associated with aging, fatigue, hair loss, infertility, and developmental issues.

Surprisingly, the appearance of your hair is tied to Kidney health in Chinese medicine. Lush, healthy hair is a sign of abundant Kidney Jing, while thinning, brittle, or prematurely graying hair may suggest a deficiency. In this view, caring for the Kidneys supports both vitality and external signs of wellness, like thick, healthy hair.

The Kidneys are also deeply connected to reproduction and fertility. They govern the development and function of the reproductive organs, influence menstrual health, and play a vital role in conception and the ability to carry a pregnancy. In men and women alike, strong Kidney energy contributes to fertility and the health of future generations.

In TCM, the Kidneys are known as the root of both Yin and Yang in the body, giving them a foundational role in maintaining internal balance. Kidney Yin provides cooling, moistening, and nourishing functions, while Kidney Yang offers warmth, activation, and motivation. When these forces are balanced, all bodily functions are in harmony. However, imbalances may lead to symptoms like night sweats, hot flashes, fatigue, cold limbs, or poor circulation – reflecting either a deficiency in Kidney Yin or Kidney Yang Deficiency — can lead to a wide range of health issues, including infertility, hormonal imbalances, cold limbs, or premature aging.

The Kidneys also control the body's water metabolism, regulating the movement and balance of all bodily fluids – including blood, sweat, tears, saliva, digestive juices, urine, sexual fluids, and menstrual blood. The Kidneys determine how much water should be retained and how much should be excreted through urination. This delicate control of fluid distribution is closely related to the health of both Kidney Yin and Yang and plays a major role in overall hydration and fluid homeostasis. When Kidney function is strong, the body maintains a proper fluid balance; when weak, it may lead to edema, frequent urination, or urinary retention.

Another key role of the Kidneys is their function in receiving and anchoring Qi, especially from the Lungs. In TCM, the Lungs send Qi downward during inhalation, and the Kidneys grasp this Qi to ensure smooth and deep breathing. When this function is impaired, symptoms like shortness of breath, asthma, or shallow breathing may occur.

The Kidneys also play a vital role in supporting bone strength and nourishing the marrow. The Kidney system helps regulate the metabolism of calcium and other essential minerals, ensuring that the bones remain strong and dense. In TCM, 'marrow' refers not only to bone marrow but also includes the brain and spinal cord. Because of this, Kidney health is closely linked to mental clarity, memory, concentration, and the integrity of the skeletal system. When Kidney energy is weak, symptoms such as dizziness, poor memory, low back or knee pain, and brittle bones may appear. The Kidneys are also responsible for producing marrow that contributes to the generation of Blood and supports immune function. When Kidney energy is balanced, the bones are stable, the mind is clear, and the body's natural defense mechanisms operate effectively.

TCM also links the Kidneys to mental and emotional resilience. They are considered the source of *willpower* and *courage*, giving us the strength to face challenges and handle stress. When the Kidneys are deficient or imbalanced, people may experience fearfulness, anxiety, or a lack of motivation. People can also feel easily discouraged or mentally fatigued with Kidney Deficiency. Supporting Kidney health helps maintain a steady mood and a clear, focused mind.

In summary, Traditional Chinese Medicine views the Kidneys as the body's powerhouse — responsible for aging, reproduction, courage, bone strength, and much more. Maintaining strong Kidney energy is considered essential for overall health, longevity, and quality of life.

Different Individuals May Experience Different Symptoms With Bumpy or Lumpy Stool

Abdominal Discomfort. This condition may come with abdominal pain in the early morning, followed by the passage of loose stools. The abdominal pain typically eases after bowel movements. Stools may contain completely undigested food. Loose stools or diarrhea can also be common, often with a sensation of urgency or incomplete elimination.

Cold Sensation. Individuals with Kidney Yang Deficiency often feel excessively cold, especially in the lower back, knees, and extremities.

Low Back Pain. A dull, achy sensation in the lower back is a common sign of Kidney weakness in TCM. The Kidneys are believed to govern the lower back, bones, and marrow, so when their energy declines, it can lead to discomfort in this area. This is often accompanied by weakness or soreness in the knees and legs, reflecting the Kidneys' role in supporting the lower body.

Fatigue. Persistent fatigue or a lack of energy is a hallmark symptom. Individuals may feel chronically tired and weak.

Frequent Urination. Kidney Yang Deficiency weakens the body's ability to hold urine, leading to increased urination — especially at night. This happens because the Kidneys lose their warming and consolidating power, making it harder to regulate fluid balance.

Weakness. Muscle weakness, particularly in the legs, may be experienced. Activities that require physical strength can become challenging.

Impotence or Infertility. Kidney Yang deficiency can lead to sexual dysfunctions like impotence, premature ejaculation, infertility or decreased sex drive in men. Women can experience irregular menstruation, infertility, or decreased libido.

Edema. Mild to moderate edema or swelling, particularly in the lower limbs, may occur due to Kidney Yang Deficiency.

Water Retention. Fluid retention and bloating can be seen, especially in the abdominal area.

Frequent Urinary Infections. Kidney Yang Deficiency can make the body more susceptible to urinary tract infections.

Pallor. The complexion may appear pale or ashen, reflecting the overall lack of warmth and vitality.

Tinnitus and Hearing Problems. Ringing in the ears and hearing difficulties can be associated with Kidney Deficiency.

Impaired Cognitive Function. Poor memory, difficulty concentrating, mental fatigue and cognitive fog may be experienced.

Emotional Symptoms. Kidney Deficiency can also affect emotional well-being, leading to feelings of fear, anxiety, nervousness, irritability and depression.

Heat Sensations. Individuals with Kidney Yin Deficiency may feel hot, especially in the palms, soles, and chest, or experiencing night sweats and hot flashes.

Dryness. Dry mouth, throat, and skin, along with a persistent feeling of thirst can occur due to Kidney Yin Deficiency.

Insomnia. Without sufficient Yin fluids to keep the body cool, individuals may have difficulty falling asleep or staying asleep. Sleep can be restless with vivid dreaming.

Constipation. Stools can be dry and difficult to pass due to a lack of Kidney Yin.

Thinner Hair. Kidney Deficiency leads to thinning or premature graying.

Self-Care and Support

Adequate Rest. Ensure you get enough rest and quality sleep. Adequate sleep is essential for replenishing energy and supporting the Kidney system.

Keep Warm. Protect yourself from cold weather and drafts, especially the lower back and lower abdomen, as the Kidneys are vulnerable to cold.

Wear Warm Clothing. Dress in layers and keep the lower back and lower abdomen well-covered in cold weather.

Regular Exercise. Engage in gentle, low-impact exercises such as Tai Chi, Qi Gong, or yoga to promote circulation and energy flow in the body.

Stress Management. Practice stress-reduction techniques such as meditation, deep breathing exercises, and relaxation to minimize the impact of chronic stress on Kidney Yang.

Acupuncture and Chinese Herbal Medicine Formulas. Consult with a qualified TCM practitioner for acupuncture treatments and personalized herbal formulas tailored to your specific pattern of Kidney Deficiency.

Stay Hydrated. Drink warm or room-temperature water and herbal teas to support hydration without taxing the digestive system.

Avoid Excessive Sexual Activity. In TCM, excessive sexual activity, including excessive masturbation depletes Kidney Yang and Yin energy. Moderation is key.

Limit Stimulants. Reduce or eliminate caffeine and alcohol, which can exacerbate heat and dryness.

Foods to Relieve Kidney Deficiency

Warm food bolster the Kidneys. Foods that are gently cooked or steamed are easier for the digestive system to process. Focus on soups and stews. Warm, nourishing soups and stews made with bone broth, root vegetables, and warming herbs like ginger and cinnamon, can be particularly beneficial for Kidney Yang Deficiency.

Garlic, ginger, and onions have warming properties and can be used in cooking to offset the cold nature of vegetables and to add flavor while supporting Kidney Yang. Most fragrant or pungent herbs and spices like cinnamon, cardamom, and cloves are Yang in nature and can be added to your meals.

Herbs to nourish Kidney Yin, strengthen Kidney Qi, and support lower back and bone health include Rehmannia Root (Sheng Di Huang), Prepared Rehmannia Root (Shu Di Huang), Asiatic Cornelian Cherry Fruit (Shan Zhu

Yu), and Gordon Euryale Seed (Qian Shi). It is best to work with a qualified TCM practitioner when using herbal formulas. For daily support, kidney-tonifying teas may include goji berries, black sesame, and Chinese yam.

Root vegetables like sweet potatoes, carrots, and parsnips are warming and grounding, making them suitable choices for Kidney Yang Deficiency.

Kidney-nourishing foods include black beans, black sesame seeds, walnuts, and bone broth. Incorporate these into your diet regularly.

Whole grains with moderate amounts of brown rice, oats, and quinoa provide sustained energy and are considered beneficial for Kidney Yang.

Barley is cooling and can be used in soups and beverages to support Kidney Yin.

Millet supports Yin and is a cooling grain that can be used as an alternative to rice.

Lean meats such as chicken, lamb, and beef are excellent sources of protein that support Kidney Yang. Fish like salmon and mackerel can also be included.

Eggs are warming and protein-rich, making them a suitable choice for Kidney Yang Deficiency.

Nuts and seeds like walnuts and black sesame seeds are considered Kidney-nourishing foods. They can be sprinkled on cereals or added to dishes.

Oysters, in small quantities, can be included in the diet. Oysters are considered a natural aphrodisiac. Sex drive is a Kidney function as the Kidneys control reproduction.

Cooked fruits, especially when lightly stewed, can be easier to digest and warming for the body. Apples, pears, and berries are good choices.

Kidney beans are named for their shape, which resembles a kidney, and are associated with supporting Kidney function.

Honey is known for its moistening properties and can be used in small amounts as a natural sweetener. The moistening quality of honey supports Yin energy.

Goji berries are considered to nourish Yin energy and can be added to teas or eaten as snacks.

Traditional Chinese herbal soups and tonics, such as ginseng chicken soup or astragalus soup, nourish Kidney Yang.

Foods that Can Worsen Kidney Deficiency

Iced drinks and cold beverages should be avoided. Opt for warm or room-temperature beverages instead.

Raw fruits and vegetables, particularly those with a cooling nature, such as watermelon, cucumber, and lettuce, can be problematic for Kidney Yang Deficiency. Watermelon is not only cooling but also a diuretic, which can increase urination and potentially weaken Kidney Yang. Cucumbers have a high water content and are considered cooling in nature. Tropical fruits like bananas and persimmons, as well as citrus fruits, can be cooling and should be consumed in moderation.

Coffee and other caffeinated beverages have a drying effect on the body. From a TCM perspective, excessive consumption can deplete Kidney Yin, which is responsible for nourishing and cooling the body. Over time, this imbalance may lead to symptoms such as restlessness, insomnia, or dryness.

Cold or raw foods, such as chilled desserts and salads, should be limited. From a TCM perspective, they are not good for Kidney Yang, as the cooling nature of these foods can further weaken the body's warming energy.

Raw seafood should be consumed sparingly, as raw fish is considered cold and damp in nature in TCM. In addition, eating raw seafood increases the risk of parasites, which can further weaken digestion and overall health.

Dairy products, especially cold milk and ice cream, can be challenging for the Spleen to digest. Fermented dairy products, such as yogurt served at room temperature, may be tolerated better by some individuals because they contain probiotics that support gut health. However, from a TCM perspective, yogurt is still considered cold in nature. This cooling quality may weaken the Spleen and Kidney Yang encourage the formation of Dampness, especially if eaten in excess or when digestion is already weak.

Sugary foods should be limited or avoided. Excessive consumption of sugary foods and beverages can weaken Kidney Yang energy.

Salty foods can exacerbate fluid imbalances and should be limited.

Soy products, such as tofu and soy milk, have a cooling effect on the body. From a TCM perspective, excessive consumption may not be ideal for individuals with Kidney Yang deficiency, since too much cooling energy can further weaken Yang.

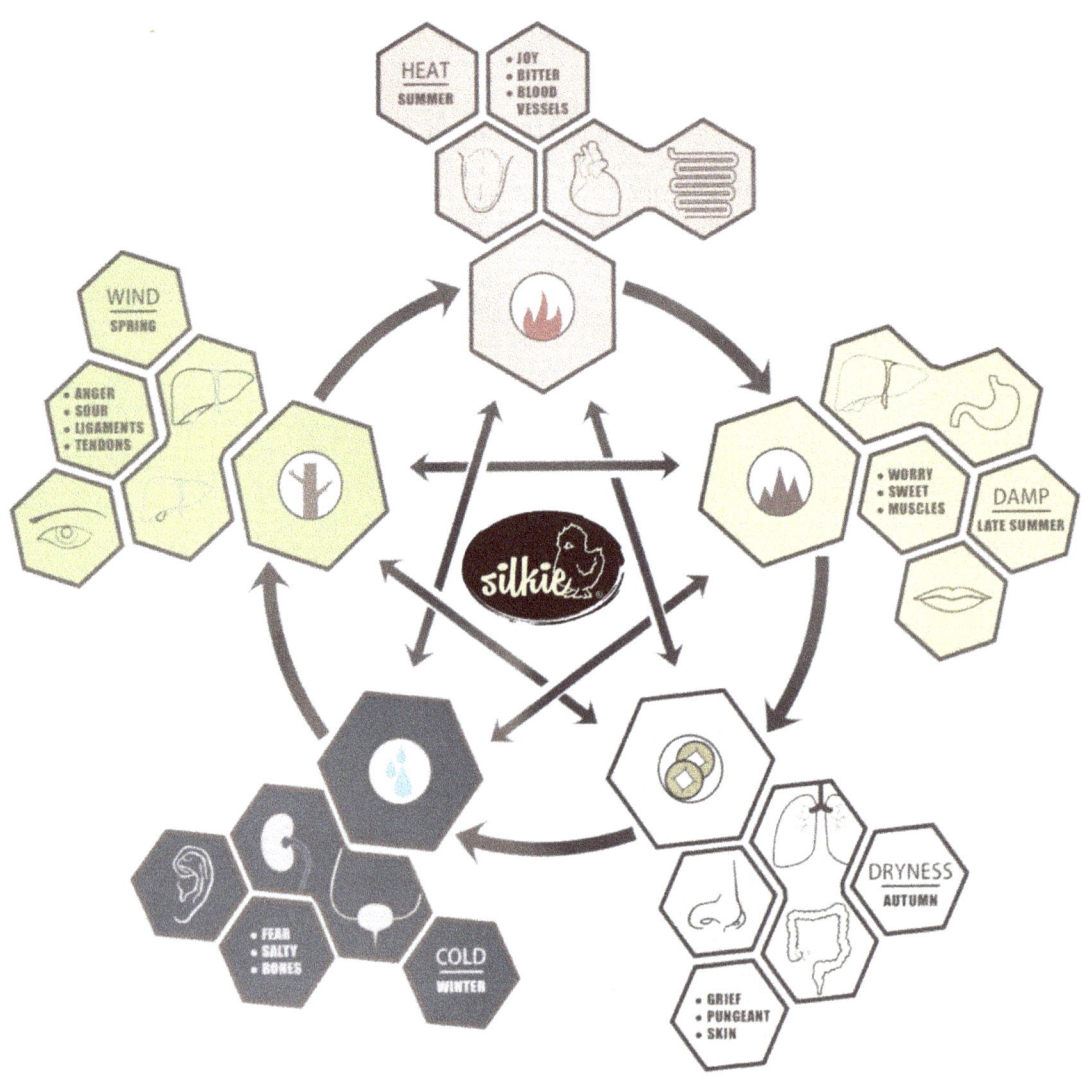

2. Dry, Dark Brown Stool with Cracks – Indicative of internal Heat

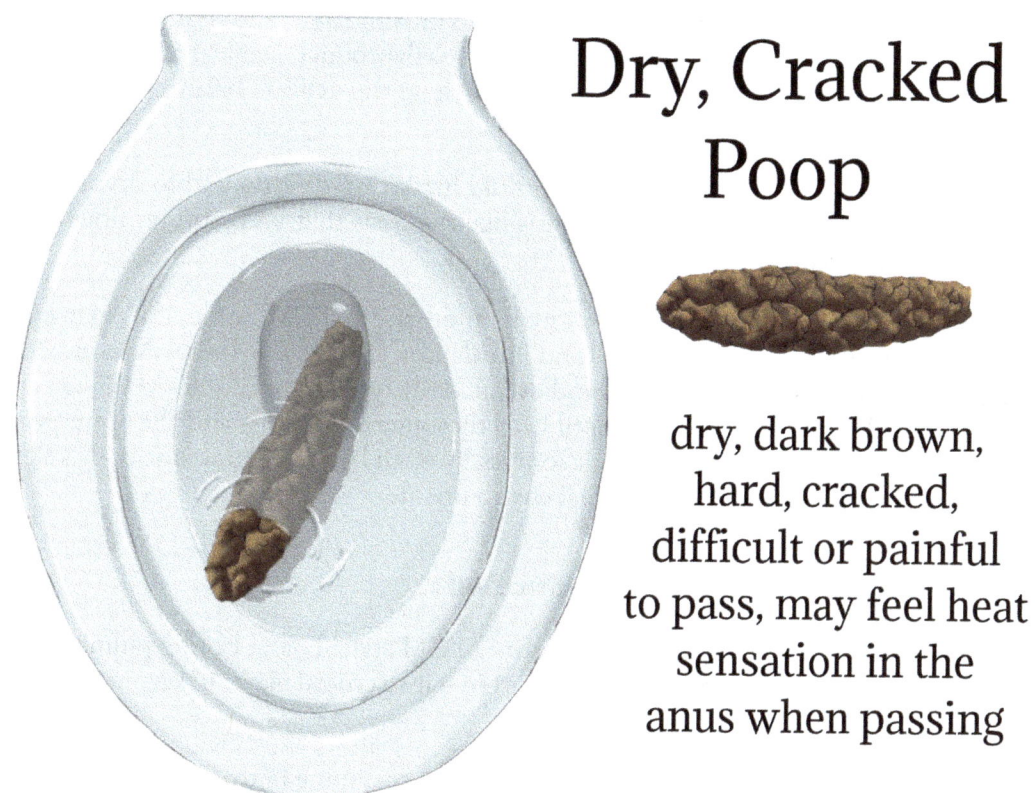

Dry, Cracked Poop

dry, dark brown, hard, cracked, difficult or painful to pass, may feel heat sensation in the anus when passing

Figure 6.2 Dry, cracks on the surface, dark brown stool, constipation, Excess Heat in the Intestines, Fluid Deficiency, Large Intestine Dryness.

What it Means: If your poop is dry and dark brown with cracks on the surface, it represents heat trapped in the Large Intestine. This condition involves dry and hard stools that are difficult to pass. You might not have bowel movements daily. Dry, cracked, dark brown stool is often a pattern of excessive heat, which can deplete the body's fluids and cause the colon to overheat.

Underlying Causes

Why might your stool be dry and dark brown? In the insightful world of Traditional Chinese Medicine, this isn't just a random occurrence; it's often a sign that things are getting a little too fiery and parched within your digestive landscape. Let's explore some of the common culprits behind this internal "heatwave."

Think of your digestive system as a delicate pot simmering on a stove. Regularly indulging in a diet that's excessively heating or spicy can turn that simmer into a rolling boil! We're talking about those delicious but fiery fried and grilled goodies, heavily spiced dishes that set your tongue tingling, and perhaps those extra cups of coffee or that nightcap that feels so relaxing. Over time, these choices can stoke the internal fires, leading to dryness and that telltale darker stool.

But it's not just about what we eat; our inner emotional world plays a significant role too. Imagine chronic stress or pent-up emotions as kindling tossed onto that digestive fire. In TCM, these imbalances can disrupt the smooth flow of Qi, our vital energy, leading to a build-up of heat in various organs, including our trusty Large Intestine. If you're the type whose digestion grinds to a halt and gets backed up under stress, that dry, dark stool might be your body's way of saying, "Things are getting a little too heated in here!"

Sometimes, the fire within isn't just from our lifestyle; it can be due to more significant internal disturbances. Conditions like Inflammatory Bowel Diseases (IBD), such as Crohn's and ulcerative colitis, are characterized by a persistent, smoldering inflammation within the digestive tract. This chronic inflammation naturally generates heat, which can manifest in those dry, darker bowel movements. Similarly, unwelcome invaders like bacterial or viral infections in our gut can ignite a fiery response, leading to inflammation and heat accumulation as our body tries to fight them off – think of it as a battleground where heat is a byproduct. Even seemingly helpful medications, especially certain antibiotics and NSAIDs, can sometimes irritate the delicate balance of our digestive system, potentially contributing to this internal heat and dryness.

Of course, just like a parched desert, a lack of sufficient fluid intake can directly lead to dryness throughout our body, including the digestive tract. Proper hydration is like the oasis that keeps things flowing smoothly and prevents that arid, dark quality in our stool.

Finally, just as some people naturally feel the cold more than others, in TCM, some of us may have an inherent constitution that makes us more prone to heat-related imbalances. It's like our internal thermostat is set a little higher from the get-go, influenced by our genetics and overall body type. So, while lifestyle choices play a big role, our inherent nature can also make us more susceptible to that internal dryness and the corresponding changes in our stool. By understanding these potential "heat sources," we can better listen to our body's signals and work towards restoring a cooler, more harmonious internal environment.

Why The Large Intestine Is Important To Our Body

Let's peek into the fascinating world of the Large Intestine, TCM style! Forget boring plumbing; in Traditional Chinese Medicine, this organ is way more than just a waste bin – it's a crucial player in keeping our inner ecosystem happy and humming!

Think of the Large Intestine as your body's savvy sanitation crew, swooping in to collect all the leftover grub after the digestive party. Its main gig is to gather up that undigested food residue and, with a bit of alchemical magic, transform it into the stuff we need to *release*. This isn't just about tidying up; it's a vital detoxification process, helping us bid farewell to unwanted guests like toxins, heavy metals, and even excess *Heat*!

Now, imagine the Large Intestine as a meticulous water wizard, expertly managing the fluid levels within our bodies. Locally, it's the gatekeeper of our bowel movements, ensuring things flow smoothly and preventing the discomfort of either a drought (constipation) or a flash flood (diarrhea). But its influence extends further, helping to maintain a harmonious balance of fluids throughout our entire system, preventing unwelcome swelling or puffiness.

But wait, there's more! Our trusty Large Intestine even moonlights as a mini internal air conditioner. In TCM, it's understood to have the power to purge excess *heat* from our system. Ever feel feverish, irritable, or maybe a little too wired? Sometimes, a good clear-out courtesy of the Large Intestine can help cool those fiery emotions and bring us back to a more even keel. It's like hitting the reset button on our internal thermostat!

Here's where things get really interesting: in TCM, our guts aren't just about processing food; they're deeply intertwined with our emotions. Think of those gut feelings – TCM takes that literally! When we're stressed, angry, or down in the dumps, it can throw the Large Intestine's rhythm out of whack. And the connection goes both ways – a grumpy Large Intestine can sometimes make us feel more emotionally volatile. A healthy Large Intestine, however, helps us practice the art of letting go, not just of physical waste, but also of thoughts and feelings that no longer serve us, allowing us to move forward with a lighter spirit.

Now, let's talk about energy highways! In TCM, the Large Intestine isn't just a standalone organ; it's one of 12 primary energy channels in the body. This Large Intestine channel has its own unique route, and by tapping into specific acupuncture points along this pathway, we can influence a whole range of health issues, far beyond just digestion. Take the famous He Gu point (LI 4) on your hand, for example – it's a go-to for tackling frontal headaches, often providing surprising relief with just gentle pressure!

Ultimately, TCM views our health as a grand, interconnected puzzle. The Large Intestine is a crucial piece, influencing and being influenced by other parts of our amazing machine. That's why a TCM practitioner might pay close attention to the state of your Large Intestine to get a broader understanding of your overall well-being. They might also peek at your tongue, feel your pulse, observe your complexion, or gently palpate different areas of your body, all in an effort to decipher the big picture of your overall health. It's all part of the fascinating detective work of TCM, where even our eliminations offer valuable insights into our inner harmony!

Different Individuals May Experience Different Symptoms With Dry, Dark Brown Stool

Constipation. Heat can dry out the stool and slow down the transit time through the Large Intestine, leading to difficulty in passing stools. Stools may be dry, hard, and difficult to eliminate.

Heat Sensation. You might notice other heat signs in the body: flushed face, red eyes, and a mild feeling of heat in your body. When your tongue looks red with a yellow and dry coating, and your pulse is rapid, it is often due to excessive heat that has affected the body's fluids and intestines. People with this pattern usually prefer cooler environments to balance the internal heat.

Dry Stools. Heat in the Large Intestine can cause stools to become dry, making bowel movements uncomfortable and potentially painful.

Abdominal Discomfort. Individuals may experience abdominal discomfort, including a feeling of heat or irritation in the abdomen. This discomfort can range from mild to moderate with a feeling of fullness, irritability, or a bloated abdomen that's sensitive to pressure. The abdominal discomfort persists or may worsen when pressure is applied to the abdomen.

Thirst and Dry Mouth. Excess heat in the Large Intestine can lead to increased thirst and a dry or sticky sensation in the mouth, a bitter taste, bad breath, and sores on the lips. People with this pattern usually prefer cold drinks to help cool the body and relieve discomfort.

Red Tongue. A red or reddish tongue with a yellow coating is commonly associated with heat patterns in TCM, including heat trapped in the Large Intestine.

Irritability and Restlessness. Heat patterns in TCM are often linked to emotional states such as irritability, restlessness, and sometimes anxiety.

Bad Breath. Excessive heat in the Large Intestine may contribute to bad breath or a foul taste in the mouth.

Skin Issues. Heat patterns can sometimes manifest on the skin, leading to conditions like a flushed face, acne, rashes, or redness, especially in the facial area.

Frequent Urination. Heat patterns may also affect the urinary system, leading to increased urination or a burning sensation during urination.

Dark or Yellow Urine. Dark or yellow urine may be an indicator of a heat pattern.

Self-Care and Support

Hydration. Stay well-hydrated by drinking plenty of water and herbal teas. Avoid coffee, caffeinated teas, and energy drinks as they are diuretics and can dry out the body. Proper hydration helps maintain balance and prevents dryness in the digestive tract.

Fiber-Rich Diet. Include fiber-rich foods like whole grains, fruits, and vegetables to support healthy digestion and regular bowel movements.

Cooling Foods to Relieve Internal Heat

Watermelon is a hydrating fruit that helps to reduce internal heat.

Cucumber contains cucurbitacins with anti-inflammatory properties and provides hydration.

Lettuce is rich in fiber and water and helps to cool the body.

Celery offers fiber and vitamins, aids in toxin removal, and supports cooling.

Coconut water is hydrating and cooling, helping to alleviate intestinal heat.

Mung beans are often used in TCM to clear heat in the body, including the intestines.

Aloe vera gel, when extracted and consumed in moderation, can have a cooling effect on the digestive system.

Chrysanthemum tea is known for its cooling properties and can help reduce heat in the body, including the intestines.

Bitter melon has a cooling nature and is used in TCM to clear heat from the digestive system.

Please note that these cooling foods should be consumed in moderation to avoid over cooling the system and creating potential digestive issues like diarrhea.

Herbs to clear Heat, moisten dryness, and promote bowel movement include Scutellaria Root (Huang Qin), Ophiopogon Tuber (Mai Dong), and Glauber's Salt (Mang Xiao). A soothing herbal tea can be made with chrysanthemum flowers and lotus leaf to gently reduce excess heat. It is best to work with a qualified TCM practitioner when using herbal formulas. For daily support, a soothing herbal tea can be made with chrysanthemum flowers and lotus leaf to gently reduce excess heat.

Foods that Can Worsen Internal Heat

Spicy foods irritate the digestive system and increase inflammation.

Heavily seasoned foods can also irritate the digestive system and contribute to inflammation.

Fried, grilled, or crunchy foods are considered "hot" because they are cooked at high temperatures and are often high in fat.

Heavy meals stress the digestive system and exacerbate internal heat.

Alcohol and coffee dehydrate the body and intensify internal heat.

3. Initial Dry and Hard Segment, Then Soft and Thinner Stool - Indicative of Spleen Qi Deficiency with Dampness/Mucus

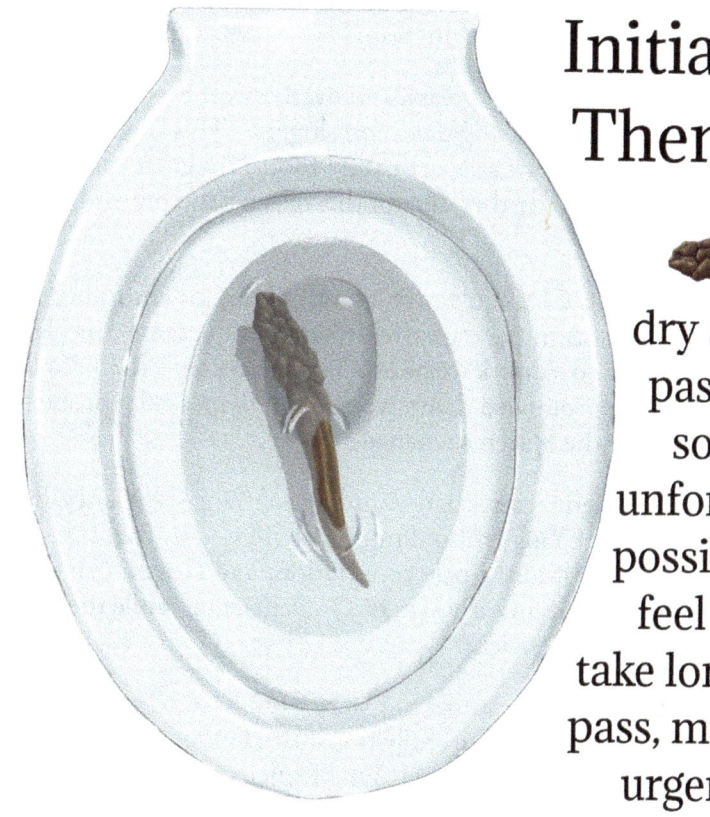

Initial Dry, Hard Then Soft Stool

dry and difficult to pass, followed by softer, loose or unformed segments, possible mucus, may feel incomplete or take longer than usual to pass, may have a sense of urgency after meals

Figure 6.3 Initial dry and hard then soft and loose stool, Spleen Qi Deficiency with Dampness and weak digestive movement.

What it Means: Have you ever noticed your stool starting off hard and dry, only to turn soft, mushy, or even loose by the end of the bowel movement? In Traditional Chinese Medicine, this isn't just a digestive quirk — it's a classic sign of Spleen Qi Deficiency with Dampness.

The Spleen plays a central role in transforming food into Qi and Blood and distributing fluids throughout the body. When the Spleen is weak, its ability to regulate fluids becomes inconsistent. At the beginning of elimination, fluids may be poorly distributed or consumed by mild Deficiency Heat, leaving the stool hard, dry, and difficult to pass. As the bowel movement continues, the weakened Spleen fails to maintain proper transformation and transportation, allowing Dampness to mix with food residue. The result is soft, unformed, or even mushy stool toward the end.

This uneven stool quality reflects a digestive system that cannot sustain balance throughout the entire process. Early dryness comes from mismanaged fluids or mild Heat, while later stool softness arises from Dampness and poor transformation. Patients often notice other symptoms such as bloating, fatigue, poor appetite, and a heavy sensation in the body — all further evidence of a weakened Spleen and sometimes a compromised Stomach.

If left unaddressed, this imbalance can worsen. Dampness may accumulate, further slowing digestion and contributing to heaviness and fatigue. In more complex cases, underlying Qi and Blood Deficiency can also give rise to Deficiency Heat, which dries out part of the stool, while poor transformation leaves the latter part soft, loose, or even containing undigested food and mucus. The hard portion may be uncomfortable and difficult to pass, while the softer portion tends to pass more easily — a frustrating cycle that clearly reflects a weakened digestive system.

Underlying Causes

In Traditional Chinese Medicine, the Spleen is seen as the body's "digestive powerhouse," responsible for transforming the food and drink we consume into Qi, Blood, and fluids, then transporting them throughout the body. When Spleen Qi is weak, this vital process slows down, leading to incomplete transformation of food and poor fluid regulation. One common sign of this weakness is stool that starts out hard and then turns soft or loose — showing the Spleen's inability to maintain consistent digestive function.

The foods we eat strongly influence Spleen health. Cold, raw, greasy, and overly sweet foods place a heavy burden on the Spleen, slowing down its transformative fire and leaving digestion sluggish. This is why someone may feel bloated, fatigued, or heavy after eating ice-cold drinks, raw salads, or fried foods. Irregular eating habits, such as skipping meals, eating on the run, or eating late at night, further disrupt the Spleen's rhythm and weaken its ability to process food.

Lifestyle and emotional stress also play major roles. Chronic worry, overthinking, or emotional strain directly injure the Spleen's Qi, much like how stress ties knots in the digestive process. At the same time, lack of physical activity prevents Qi from circulating smoothly, while overwork without adequate rest depletes the Spleen's reserves. Living in damp environments or being exposed to prolonged damp weather can worsen the problem, as external Dampness seeps inward, creating a heavier load for the Spleen to manage.

If this weakness continues for years, Spleen Qi Deficiency can progress into Spleen Yang Deficiency. In this case, not only is Qi weak, but the warming, activating force of Yang is also diminished. This adds cold signs to the picture — cold hands and feet, loose stools with undigested food, a pale complexion, and fatigue that worsens in cold environments. The hard-then-soft stool pattern may be an early sign of Qi Deficiency, while the presence of cold symptoms suggests the Spleen's Yang has also become deficient.

Understanding these underlying causes helps explain why stools can shift from hard to soft in the same bowel movement. It reflects a digestive system that lacks the strength to fully transform food from beginning to end — a hallmark of weakened Spleen Qi, and in more advanced cases, Spleen Yang Deficiency.

Why The Spleen Is Important To Our Body

In the rich tapestry of Traditional Chinese Medicine, the Spleen holds a place of profound importance, far beyond its Western anatomical counterpart. Here, it's considered the absolute cornerstone of your digestive system, a bustling hub encompassing the functions of the pancreas and more. Its main mission? To skillfully transform every bite of food and sip of fluid into the vital energy known as Qi and the nourishing substance called Blood. These two powerhouses, Qi and Blood, then become the very lifeblood, literally, that fuels and sustains every organ and tissue in your body. Think of it as the ultimate internal alchemist, ensuring you extract every last drop of energy and nutrient from what you consume.

The Spleen is often hailed as the primary producer of what TCM calls "postnatal Qi" – the energy we derive directly from our food. This isn't just a small boost; this postnatal Qi is what powers all your daily activities, from deep thinking to vigorous exercise, and critically, it's what helps your body fend off illness. While the Liver traditionally handles the storage and regulation of Blood, the Spleen plays a crucial supporting role in both its production and overall quality. A healthy Spleen means healthy Blood, which in turn means your muscles, organs, and every single cell are properly nourished and ready for action. Once the Spleen has worked its magic, transforming food into Qi and Blood, it then takes on the vital role of distributing these essential substances throughout your entire system. It's like the body's internal shipping company, ensuring every organ – from the Heart and Lungs to the Kidneys – receives the precious nourishment and Qi it needs to function optimally.

But the Spleen's influence doesn't stop there! It directly impacts your muscle and limb strength. If you've ever seen someone with soft, flabby muscles, in TCM, that often points to a weakened Spleen. Conversely, a strong Spleen is the secret behind physical endurance and the effortless ability to move through your day. Your immune system also heavily relies on a robust Spleen. By efficiently converting food into the energy and Blood that supports all bodily systems, a healthy Spleen essentially acts as the immune system's primary fuel station, empowering it to stand strong against invaders.

The Spleen even has a unique "holding" or "lifting" function in TCM. The Spleen is responsible for keeping your organs in their proper place. If an organ starts to sag or prolapse – like a uterine prolapse, for instance – it's often a telltale sign of a weakened Spleen unable to maintain its upward-supporting energy.

Finally, a healthy, balanced Spleen is deeply connected to a calm and stable mind. When the Spleen's harmony is disturbed, you might find yourself caught in endless "looping thoughts," or experience emotional disturbances like excessive worry and overthinking. It's a powerful reminder of how intricately our physical well-being is linked to our mental and emotional states in TCM.

Different Individuals May Experience Different Symptoms With Dry and Hard, Then Soft and Thinner Stool

Digestive Issues. The Spleen plays a central role in digestion, so digestive symptoms are common. These may include bloating, abdominal distension, loose stools or diarrhea (with undigested food particles), poor appetite, and a feeling of fullness in the abdomen, particularly after eating.

Fatigue. Spleen Yang Deficiency can lead to a lack of energy and generalized fatigue. Individuals may feel physically and mentally exhausted. Individuals with Spleen Qi deficiency often experience low energy levels and persistent fatigue. This fatigue may be physical and/or mental, leading to a sense of heaviness and sluggishness.

Cold Sensitivity. Spleen Yang Deficiency is associated with a lack of warmth in the body. As a result, individuals may experience sensitivity to cold temperatures, cold limbs, and a preference for warm environments and foods. They might feel chilled easily and have a hard time warming up.

Edema. Spleen Yang Deficiency can result in the accumulation of dampness (unhealthy fluid) in the body. This may manifest as edema, particularly in the lower extremities. Edema is characterized by swelling and fluid retention.

Excessive Phlegm. Besides edema, dampness accumulation can also lead to the formation of phlegm in the body. This can result in symptoms such as phlegm in the throat, a sensation of fullness in the chest, and a tendency to cough up mucus. It may also cause the formation of painless, doughy lumps found under the skin.

Weakened Immunity. The Spleen Yang Deficiency can weaken the body's immune system, making individuals more susceptible to illnesses and infections. They may experience frequent colds and infections.

Mental Dullness. TCM associates the Spleen with the mind, particularly clear thinking and concentration. Spleen Yang Deficiency may result in mental fog, forgetfulness, and difficulty concentrating.

Weight Gain. Due to impaired metabolism and digestion, some individuals with Spleen Yang Deficiency may start to crave sweets as a source of quick energy. This craving for sweets can interfere with weight management and cause weight gain.

Reproductive Issues. Spleen Yang Deficiency can affect the reproductive system, leading to irregular menstruation, fertility problems, or excessive vaginal discharge, especially in women.

Excessive Discharge. Leukorrhea (abnormal vaginal discharge) is a form of excess mucus that has accumulated due to poor functioning of the Spleen. Leukorrhea is common among women who eat a lot of sweets.

Poor Appetite. Spleen Yang Deficiency can lead to a reduced appetite and a lack of interest in food. Individuals may have difficulty maintaining a healthy appetite.

Bruising and Easy Bleeding. Weakened Spleen Qi can affect blood clotting, leading to easy bruising and prolonged bleeding from minor injuries or cuts.

Frequent Urination. Spleen Yang Deficiency can lead to increased urination and pale urine.

Pale Complexion. A pale or sallow complexion often reflects insufficient Blood supply due to Spleen Qi Deficiency. When the Spleen cannot transform food into Qi and Blood effectively, the skin lacks proper nourishment and loses its natural glow.

Tongue and Pulse Signs. In TCM diagnosis, a pale tongue with a thin, white coating and a deep, weak pulse are characteristic signs of Spleen Yang Deficiency.

Self-Care and Support

Chew Thoroughly. Chew your food thoroughly to aid the digestive process.

Exercise Moderately. Engage in gentle, regular exercise like walking, tai chi, or yoga to promote circulation and overall well-being.

Manage Stress. Stress can weaken Spleen function. Practice stress-reduction techniques such as meditation or deep breathing exercises.

Get Adequate Rest. Ensure you get enough rest and sleep. Rest is essential for replenishing Qi.

Stay Warm. Protect yourself from cold and damp environments, especially during colder seasons.

Get Professional Help. Consult a qualified TCM practitioner for herbal formulas tailored to your specific Spleen deficiency pattern. Common herbs used for Spleen deficiency include ginseng, licorice root, and astragalus. Additionally, acupuncture treatments can help restore balance to the Spleen.

Avoid Self-Diagnosis. It's essential to consult a licensed TCM practitioner for a proper diagnosis and personalized treatment plan. Spleen deficiency can manifest differently in individuals, and treatment should be tailored to your specific condition.

Be Patient and Consistent. TCM treatments often require time and consistent effort. Be patient with the process, and follow your practitioner's guidance diligently.

Eat Regular Meals. Establish a routine of eating three balanced meals a day at consistent times (7 am, 12 pm, and 5 pm) to support the Spleen's function.

Avoid Overeating. Stop eating before you feel overly full. Undereating slightly is better than overeating, as it avoids straining the digestive system.

Skip Late-Night Eating. Allow at least 2.5 hours between your last meal and bedtime to aid digestion. It is best not to eat after 7 pm.

Foods To Relieve Spleen Yang Deficiency

Cooked foods are easier to digest than raw foods and are gentler on the Spleen. To invigorate your Spleen Yang, prioritize warming foods prepared with cooking methods like slow cooking, simmering, or steaming, as these processes infuse dishes with beneficial warm energy. Focus on soups, stews, and cooked vegetables.

Pungent spices such as ginger, cinnamon, garlic, onions, and black pepper also add Yang energy to foods.

Root vegetables are grounding and have a warming effect on the body. Potatoes, sweet potatoes, carrots, and parsnips can be beneficial.

Whole grains like rice, oats, quinoa, and barley provide sustained energy and are nourishing for the Spleen. Avoid excessive consumption of refined grains and processed foods.

Lean meats are warming and provide essential amino acids for energy and tissue repair. Small, regular portions of animal protein can support the Spleen. Chicken and turkey are good options.

Healthy fats like olive oil, avocados, and nuts can be incorporated into your diet for overall nourishment.

Herbs to strengthen the Spleen, resolve Dampness, and regulate fluid transformation include Codonopsis Root (Dang Shen), Poria (Fu Ling), Atractylodes Rhizome (Bai Zhu), and Tangerine Peel (Chen Pi). You can also incorporate supportive foods like Chinese yam, lotus seeds, and jujubes (red dates). It is best to work with a qualified TCM practitioner when using herbal formulas. For daily support, herbal teas can include Chinese yam, lotus seeds, and jujubes (red dates), sometimes with ginger to gently warm the Spleen.

Aromatic vegetables like garlic, onion, and leeks can enhance the flavor of dishes and support the Spleen.

Warm beverages like herbal teas made from Qi-tonifying herbs such as ginseng or astragalus can complement your diet. Ginger, lemon, and warm water are also helpful for supporting the Spleen's digestive functions when Spleen Qi is weak.

Small, frequent meals throughout the day are better than large meals This can help prevent overloading the Spleen and support better digestion.

Honey, in moderation, is beneficial for the Spleen as well as the Kidneys.

Nuts and seeds like almonds and pumpkin seeds are warming and can be added to cereals or used as snacks.

Foods That Can Worsen Spleen Yang Deficiency

Cold foods and beverages, such as salads and iced drinks, should be minimized or avoided. Cold foods and drinks diminish Yang energy and impair the Spleen's ability to transform and transport food efficiently.

Icy or frozen foods, such as popsicles, ice cold drinks, and smoothies made with frozen fruits or ice cubes, are particularly detrimental to Spleen Yang. They can slow down digestion and impair the digestive process.

Raw foods, including raw vegetables and fruits, are considered harder for the Spleen to process. Cooking or lightly steaming these foods can make them easier to digest. While fruits are nutritious, excessive consumption of raw fruits, especially tropical fruits like watermelon and pineapple, can weaken the Spleen.

Raw salads when eaten daily or in large quantities, especially in cold weather, can deplete Spleen Yang. Opt for warm, cooked vegetables instead.

Dairy products, especially cold milk and ice cream, can be challenging for the Spleen to digest. Fermented dairy products, such as yogurt served at room temperature, may be tolerated better by some individuals because they contain probiotics that support gut health. However, from a TCM perspective, yogurt is still considered cold in nature. This cooling quality may weaken the Spleen and encourage the formation of Dampness, especially if eaten when digestion is already weak.

Sugary foods and sweets can weaken the Spleen's function. This includes refined sugars, candies, and sweet beverages.

Heavy, greasy foods like deep-fried or fast food can burden the Spleen and further impair its function. Even stir-fried vegetables that are too greasy can be hard on the Spleen.

Caffeine and alcohol are "hot" in nature and can contribute to further Spleen deficiency. Foods and drinks that are hot in nature have a dehydrating effect on the body, which is counterproductive to the body's need for adequate fluids. These beverages should be consumed in moderation or avoided.

Iced teas with boba are not suitable for individuals with Spleen Yang Deficiency. As mentioned above, ice drinks dampen Yang energy. Boba is very hard to digest and sugary which will weaken the Spleen. Opt for warm or room-temperature herbal teas.

Green tea is considered cooling in TCM. Green tea has a cold and damp effect on the body. Some compounds in tea, like tannins, can inhibit the activity of digestive enzymes. This can interfere with the Spleen's ability to break down and absorb nutrients from food effectively. Digestive function is already compromised in Spleen Yang Deficiency, so it is best to avoid or minimize tea intake. Tea contains caffeine, a stimulant, so it may provide a temporary energy boost. However, this stimulant effect can further weaken Spleen's Yang energy in the long run, leading to increased fatigue and a reliance on external stimulants.

4. Finger-Like Stool Pieces - Indicative of malnutrition

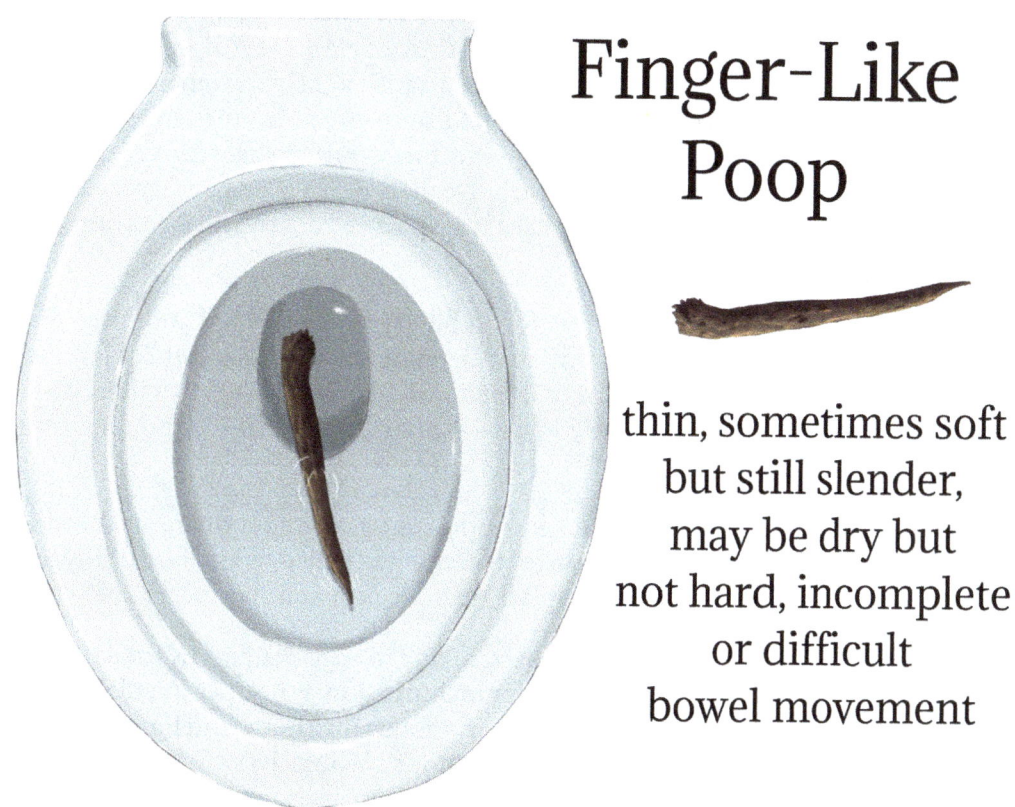

Finger-Like Poop

thin, sometimes soft but still slender, may be dry but not hard, incomplete or difficult bowel movement

Figure 6.4 Finger-like stool, Liver Qi Stagnation affecting the Spleen, Qi Deficiency or emotional stress constricting the intestines, resulting in narrow, slender stool.

What it Means: If your stool appears in thin, finger-like pieces, it is a sign of malnutrition. In Western medicine, this shape can sometimes raise concerns about spasms or narrowing of the intestinal tract, but in TCM, it's more commonly linked to stress or stagnant Qi flow. The body's Qi — especially Liver and Spleen — is not moving harmoniously. Liver Qi stagnation affecting the Spleen, can lead to poor form and shape of stool. Qi deficiency or emotional stress constricting the intestines can result in narrow, slender stool. The thin shape may also reflect weak intestinal tone or muscle that fails to push out a fuller stool. People who commonly get finger-like stool usually have poor eating habits (irregular meals) or dietary restrictions such as vegetarian, fasting or juicing diets that cause an imbalance of Yin and Yang. Additionally those who are sedentary or have suppressed emotions can also be prone to finger-like poop.

Underlying Causes

Ever wonder how something as fundamental as nourishment can go wrong? Malnutrition isn't just about not having enough food; it's a tangled web of factors that can leave the body depleted or out of balance. Think of it like this: our bodies are incredible machines that need the right fuel – calories for energy, macronutrients (proteins, fats, carbs) for structure and function, and micronutrients (vitamins and minerals) for all the intricate processes. When this fuel supply is inadequate or imbalanced, things start to break down.

Imagine trying to build a house with missing bricks or faulty wiring – that's what happens when we don't get enough of the essentials. This can be a direct result of struggles with access, where poverty or remote locations limit the availability of food. Or, it can sneak into our lives through dietary habits that consistently favor empty calories over nutrient-rich choices – think of a diet heavy on processed snacks and fast food. It's like trying to run a high-performance car on cheap, low-grade gasoline! Sometimes, the issue isn't what we eat, but what our bodies can actually *use*. Conditions like celiac disease, Crohn's, IBS, or food allergies can throw a wrench in the digestive process, hindering the absorption of vital nutrients. It's like having a leaky fuel line in that amazing machine of ours.

Then there are the health challenges that can dramatically shift our nutritional needs or sap our resources. Chronic illnesses such as cancer, diabetes, kidney disease, and HIV/AIDS often act like energy vampires, increasing the body's demands or making it harder to hold onto precious nutrients. On the other end of the spectrum, eating disorders like anorexia, bulimia, and binge-eating disorder create a battlefield with food, leading to severe nutritional deficits through restrictive diets or harmful compensatory behaviors. Even well-intentioned surgeries, like gastric bypass, can have unexpected consequences on nutrient absorption, requiring a whole new approach to eating.

But it's not just about physical health; our lifestyles play a big part too. Alcohol and drug abuse can lead to a downward spiral of poor food choices and a body that struggles to absorb and use what little nutrition it gets. And let's not forget the powerful connection between mind and body — mental health conditions like depression, anxiety, and dementia can significantly impact appetite, eating habits, and even the motivation to prepare a healthy meal.

As we journey through life, our bodies change, and aging brings its own set of nutritional hurdles. Metabolism can slow down, appetite might wane, dental issues can make eating a challenge, and our ability to absorb certain nutrients can diminish. It's like the machine needing a little more care and specialized fuel as it gets older.

Zooming out, the world around us has a profound impact. Living in areas plagued by food deserts, contaminated water, or poor sanitation creates a breeding ground for malnutrition, especially in vulnerable communities. Socioeconomic factors like poverty, famine, lack of education about nutrition, and limited access to healthcare form a powerful undercurrent that erodes our ability to nourish ourselves. Even economic and political instability can send shockwaves through food supply chains, leaving entire regions vulnerable to shortages.

Zooming in, parasitic infections can cause malnutrition. Imagine tiny, unwelcome guests setting up shop inside your body — that's what happens with parasites! These sneaky invaders can steal the very nutrients you eat, like they're dipping into your dinner plate before you even get a chance. Some can even cause tummy troubles that make it hard to digest food properly, meaning you're not getting all the good stuff you need. Over time, this constant nutrient theft and digestive disruption can leave you feeling weak, tired, and yes, malnourished, because your body isn't getting the fuel it needs to thrive.

Finally, even things we might not immediately connect to nutrition can play a role. Certain medications and medications for weight loss can have sneaky side effects, interfering with how our bodies absorb and use nutrients. And those extreme diets or rapid weight loss trends — like juice cleanses, the HCG diet, very low-calorie diets (VLCDs) such as the 800-calorie diet, long-term fasting, or poorly planned vegan diets — can backfire spectacularly, leading to serious nutritional deficiencies if not approached with proper knowledge and expert guidance.

Malnutrition isn't a simple problem with a single cause. It's a complex story woven from our individual choices, our health, our environment, and the broader societal forces at play. Understanding these interconnected pieces is key to tackling this widespread challenge.

How Malnutrition Can Affect Our Body

In the vibrant tapestry of Traditional Chinese Medicine, nourishment isn't just about calories; it's about cultivating the vital energies and precious substances that animate our entire being, from the strength in our muscles to the harmony within our organs and the clarity of our minds. When this fundamental nourishment falters, like a flame starved of fuel, the very foundation of our well-being is undermined.

Imagine your body's energy, or Qi, as a vibrant current flowing through you, the very spark of life. Malnutrition acts like a drain on this current, leading to a deficiency. When Qi is low, that get-up-and-go vanishes, leaving you feeling perpetually tired and lacking your usual zest for life.

TCM also speaks of Blood, not just as the crimson tide within us, but as a rich reservoir of the nutrients that sustain every cell. When malnutrition sets in, this vital Blood becomes insufficient, leaving its mark with telltale signs like pale skin, a dizzying lightness of the head, and a Heart that races as if trying to compensate for the shortage.

Harmony is the cornerstone of TCM, the delicate dance between Yin and Yang, the opposing yet complementary forces within us. Malnutrition can disrupt this elegant balance, tipping the scales and causing you to feel excessively hot (a Yang imbalance) or perpetually cold (a Yin imbalance). This disharmony can manifest in various ways, from feeling parched and overheated to experiencing persistent dryness.

Think of your internal organs – the Spleen diligently transforming food into energy, the Liver ensuring smooth flow, and the Kidneys as the root of our vital essence – as a well-orchestrated team. Malnutrition weakens these crucial players, particularly the Spleen's digestive power, leading to a chorus of tummy troubles and inefficient nutrient absorption.

Furthermore, when nourishment is lacking, the smooth flow of Qi and Blood can become sluggish and stagnant, like a dry streambed. This stagnation can manifest as nagging abdominal pain, unpredictable bowel movements, and a general feeling of discomfort and obstruction within the body.

The impact of malnutrition extends beyond the physical realm, reaching into the landscape of our emotions and thoughts. Just as a plant withers without water, our minds can become hazy and our spirits shriveled by a lack of nourishment. This can manifest as feelings of sadness that linger, anxieties that gnaw, or a general irritability that casts a shadow over our days.

Our body's defense system, akin to a vigilant guardian, also relies heavily on proper nourishment. Malnutrition weakens the immune system, leaving us more vulnerable to the attacks of external pathogens and making us more susceptible to common colds and persistent infections.

The most concerning aspect of prolonged malnutrition in TCM is its capacity to deeply deplete our fundamental energies and vital substances – the Qi, Blood, Yin, and Yang that are the very building blocks of our health. Over time, this profound depletion can lead to serious and enduring health issues, casting a long shadow over our well-being. Just as a garden left untended withers into dust and silence, so too does the body when starved of nourishment, loses its resilience and the quiet flame of its vitality.

Different Individuals May Experience Different Symptoms With Finger-Like Stool

Fatigue. Feeling excessively tired and lacking energy is a common symptom of malnutrition.

Weakness. Muscle weakness and a general lack of strength can occur due to nutrient deficiencies.

Weight Loss. Unintended and significant weight loss can be a noticeable sign of malnutrition.

Pale or Dry Skin. Malnutrition can lead to changes in skin color and texture, making the skin appear pale, dry, or flaky.

Hair and Nail Problems. Brittle hair, hair loss, and brittle or spoon-shaped nails (koilonychia) can be indicative of malnutrition.

Dizziness. Feeling lightheaded or dizzy may result from poor nutrient intake.

Difficulty Concentrating. Malnutrition can affect cognitive function, making it hard to concentrate and think clearly.

Depression. Changes in nutrient levels can impact mood and contribute to feelings of sadness or depression.

Digestive Problems. Malnutrition may cause digestive issues such as diarrhea, constipation, or abdominal pain. May also lead to gastrointestinal disorders, including gastritis, ulcers, and impaired nutrient absorption.

Weakened Immune System. A compromised immune system can lead to an increased susceptibility to infections.

Delayed Wound Healing. Wounds and injuries may take longer to heal in individuals with malnutrition.

Swelling. Edema, or swelling of the body, can occur, particularly in areas like the ankles and feet.

Changes in Heart Rate and Blood Pressure. Malnutrition can affect Heart rate and blood pressure, leading to irregularities.

Brittle Bones. Malnutrition can weaken bones, increasing the risk of fractures.

Anemia. A lack of essential nutrients, particularly iron and vitamins like B12 and folate, can result in anemia, characterized by fatigue, pale skin, and shortness of breath.

Hormonal Imbalances. Malnutrition can disrupt hormonal balance, potentially affecting menstrual cycles and fertility.

Impaired Growth (in children). Children with malnutrition may experience stunted growth and delayed development.

Impaired Growth (in adults). Malnutrition in adults may lead to muscle wasting and exacerbate existing muscle weakness.

Self-Care and Support

Root Cause Identification. Determine why malnutrition occurred. It could be due to inadequate food intake, digestive issues, chronic illnesses, or other factors. Addressing the root cause is crucial.

Medical Evaluation. Consult with a healthcare professional to assess the extent of malnutrition and any associated health complications. A thorough evaluation can guide treatment.

Nutritional Assessment. A registered dietitian or nutritionist can conduct a nutritional assessment to identify specific nutrient deficiencies and create a personalized nutrition plan.

Balanced Diet. Adopt a well-balanced diet that includes a variety of foods from all food groups. Emphasize fruits, vegetables, lean proteins, whole grains, and healthy fats.

Supplementation. In some cases, nutritional supplements may be necessary to address severe deficiencies. Supplements made from whole foods contain natural vitamins and minerals that are more easily digested and absorbed than synthetic vitamins and nutrients. Consult a healthcare provider for guidance.

Nutrient and Caloric Adequacy. Ensure that daily nutrient and caloric intake meets individual needs, taking into account age, gender, activity level, and health status. Adequate nutrient and caloric intake is essential for overall health.

Protein Intake. Protein is vital for tissue repair and overall health. Include sources of high-quality protein (lean meats, poultry, fish, and egg products) in the diet for each meal.

Micronutrients. Pay attention to micronutrients (vitamins and minerals) that may be deficient, such as iron, vitamin D, vitamin B12, and folic acid. Adjust the diet to include foods rich in these nutrients.

Hydration. Proper hydration is essential for nutrient absorption and overall well-being. Consume an adequate amount of water throughout the day.

Small, Frequent Meals. Eating smaller, more frequent meals can be helpful for individuals with reduced appetite or digestive issues. This approach provides a steady supply of nutrients.

Nutrition Education. Educate individuals and caregivers about proper nutrition, meal planning, and portion control to prevent malnutrition from recurring.

Monitoring and Follow-Up. Regularly monitor progress and nutrient levels through medical check-ups and nutritional assessments. Adjust the nutrition plan as needed.

Psychological Support. Address any psychological factors contributing to malnutrition, such as eating disorders or depression. Psychological support and counseling may be necessary.

Home Modifications. Ensure a safe and supportive home environment, especially for older adults, to prevent accidents and facilitate access to nutritious food.

Community Resources. Access community programs, food assistance, and social services that can provide additional support, particularly for those facing financial or logistical challenges.

Medication Management. For individuals with underlying medical conditions, managing medications as prescribed is essential to improve health and nutritional status.

Exercise and Physical Activity. Encourage appropriate physical activity to support overall health and well-being, as long as it aligns with medical recommendations.

Foods To Relieve Malnutrition

Lean meats. Chicken, turkey, pork, or small amounts of lean cuts of beef are powerhouses of high-quality protein essential for rebuilding tissues and providing energy.

Fish with fins and scales. Salmon, tuna, mackerel, and sardines are a few common examples of fish that offer easily digestible protein and beneficial omega-3 fatty acids crucial for overall health and reducing inflammation.

Eggs. Eggs are a remarkably complete food, packed with protein, healthy fats, and a wide array of vitamins and minerals vital for recovery.

Legumes. Beans, lentils, and chickpeas provide a robust combination of plant-based protein, fiber, and complex carbohydrates for sustained energy and digestive health.

Fruits and vegetables. As a collective, fruits and vegetables deLiver a broad spectrum of vitamins, minerals, and antioxidants critical for bodily functions and immune support.

Colorful fruits. The vibrant hues of fruits like berries, citrus, and kiwi indicate a rich concentration of vitamins and antioxidants that protect cells and boost immunity.

Leafy greens. Spinach, kale, Swiss chard are nutrient-dense champions, supplying essential vitamins, minerals, and fiber for healthy blood and strong bones.

Vegetables. Broccoli, carrots, and sweet potatoes are commonly available at the market and offer a diverse range of vitamins, minerals, and complex carbohydrates, supporting energy production and overall vitality.

Whole grains. Brown rice, white rice, quinoa, and oats provide sustained energy through complex carbohydrates and offer essential B vitamins for metabolism.

Whole wheat pasta. This provides complex carbohydrates and fiber, supporting steady energy and digestive regularity. However, modern wheat has been heavily hybridized and can be difficult to digest, often contributing to Dampness in those with weak Spleen Qi. If you're sensitive to wheat or gluten, consider alternatives like brown rice pasta, buckwheat soba, quinoa pasta, or spelt — an older grain that's less modified and often easier on digestion.

Whole grain bread. A good source of complex carbohydrates and dietary fiber, whole grain bread delivers sustained energy and supports gut health.

Nuts and seeds. Almonds, walnuts, Brazil nuts, chia seeds, flaxseeds, and pumpkin seeds are nutrient-rich and can strengthen the body when used keep the total around 1 teaspoon of seeds or 3–5 nut pieces daily. They provide healthy fats, protein, and minerals, but in TCM they are considered heavy and Dampness-forming if consumed in excess.

Healthy fats. Olive oil and avocado oil do provide concentrated energy and help absorb fat-soluble vitamins, but in TCM, too much oily food contributes to Dampness and sluggish digestion. A healthy amount is about 1–2 tablespoons (15–30 ml) per day total from cooking and dressing combined. This is usually enough to get the benefits without overburdening the Spleen and Stomach.

Nutrient-rich soups and stews. Soups made with a variety of vegetables, lean protein, and whole grains can provide a wealth of nutrients. Some TCM herbal soups made with a silkie chicken help to nourish the Blood and Qi.

Herbs. Herbs to tonify Qi, Blood, and improve nutrient absorption include Codonopsis Root (Dang Shen), Poria (Fu Ling), Angelica Root (Dang Gui), and Goji Berries (Gou Qi Zi). It is best to work with a qualified TCM practitioner when using herbal formulas. For daily support, a mild herbal tea with astragalus, longan fruit, and red dates supports nutrient absorption and energy.

Water, clear broths, and herbal teas. It's important to stay hydrated with liquids that can replenish you.

Supplements (Under Medical Supervision). In some cases, healthcare professionals may recommend dietary supplements to address specific nutrient deficiencies.

Foods That Can Worsen Malnutrition

Processed foods often lack essential nutrients and may be high in added sugars, unhealthy fats, and salt. Examples include sugary cereals, chips, and most fast food.

Sugary snacks and desserts such as candies, pastries, and sugary beverages provide empty calories and can displace more nutritious foods.

Fried foods like french fries and fried chicken are typically high in unhealthy fats and low in essential nutrients.

Soda and sugary drinks provide little to no nutritional value and can lead to reduced appetite for healthier foods.

Dairy products, especially cold milk and ice cream, can be challenging for the Spleen to digest. Fermented dairy products, such as yogurt served at room temperature, may be tolerated better by some individuals because they contain probiotics that support gut health. However, from a TCM perspective, yogurt is still considered cold in nature.This cooling quality may weaken the Spleen and encourage the formation of Dampness, especially if eaten when digestion is already weak. In cases of malnutrition or Spleen Qi deficiency, dairy can further strain the digestive system and hinder nutrient absorption. Full-fat dairy products can also be high in saturated fats, which may not be suitable for individuals with weak digestion, as they are harder to break down and can add extra burden to the Spleen and Stomach.

Coffee and caffeinated beverages suppress the appetite. Caffeine can interfere with nutrient absorption and may contribute to reduced caloric intake if consumed in excess.

Excessive alcohol consumption can disrupt digestion, impair nutrient absorption, and lead to poor dietary choices.

Refined carbohydrates like white bread, and sugary cereals lack fiber and essential nutrients.

High-sodium foods such as processed meats, canned soups, and many fast foods can contribute to water retention and negatively affect overall health.

Full-fat dairy products can be high in saturated fats, which may not be suitable for individuals with weak digestion.

Raw or undercooked foods can pose a risk of foodborne illnesses, which can further compromise nutrient absorption.

High-fiber and low-calorie foods, such as broccoli, cauliflower, bell peppers, zucchini, cabbage, lettuce, celery, and cucumber should be eaten in moderation. When eaten in large quantities, high fiber and low calorie foods can actually weaken the digestive system (particularly the Spleen in TCM). With malnutrition, it is important to eat more protein and less vegetables. Less is not zero!

Spicy foods and heavily seasoned dishes may irritate the digestive system and reduce appetite.

Low-nutrient foods should be limited or avoided. Filling up on foods with little nutritional value, like crackers or rice cakes, leaves little room for nutrient-rich options.

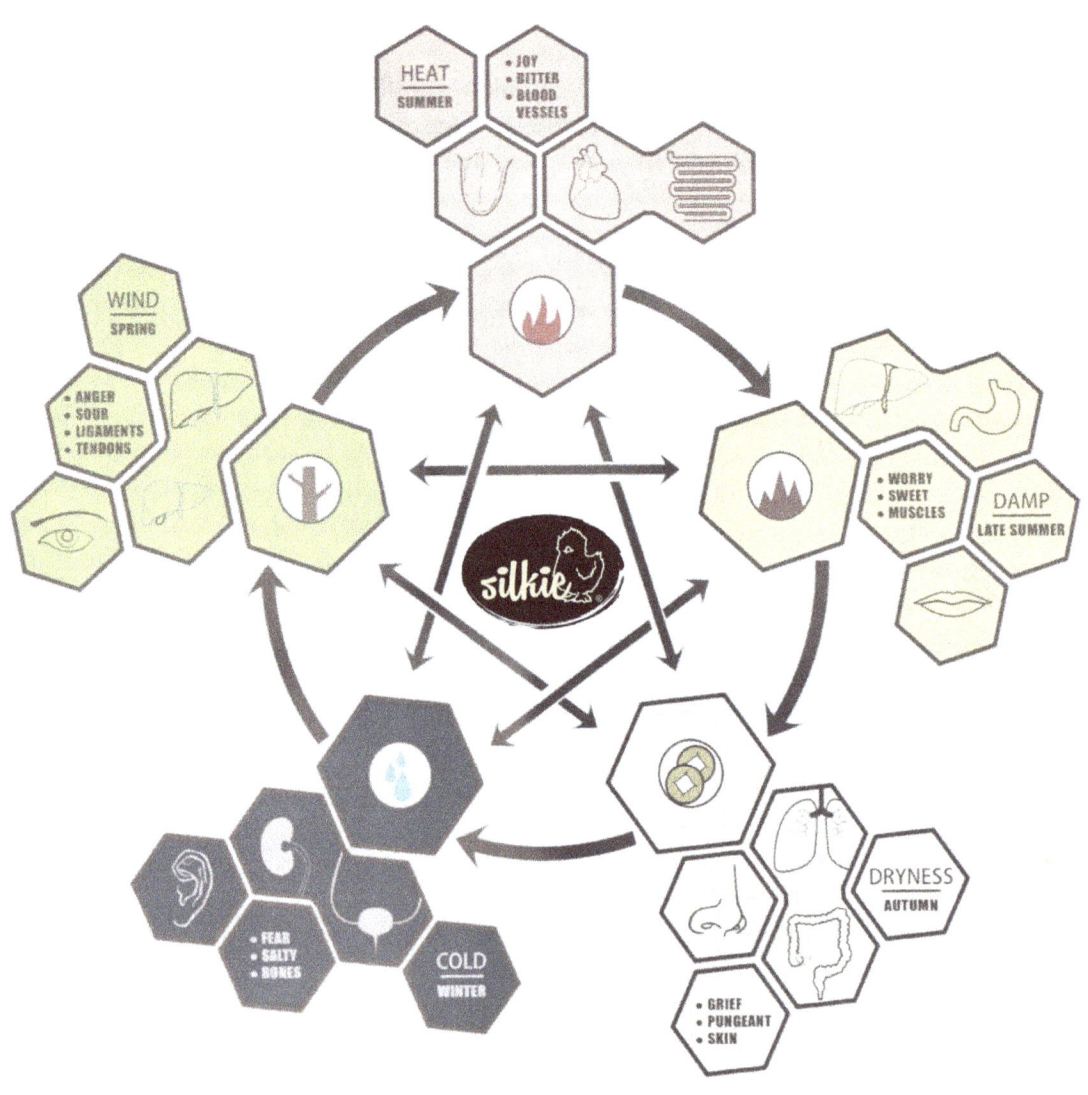

5. Fluffy Stool Pieces that are Mushy, Loose, or Soft - Liver & Spleen disharmony

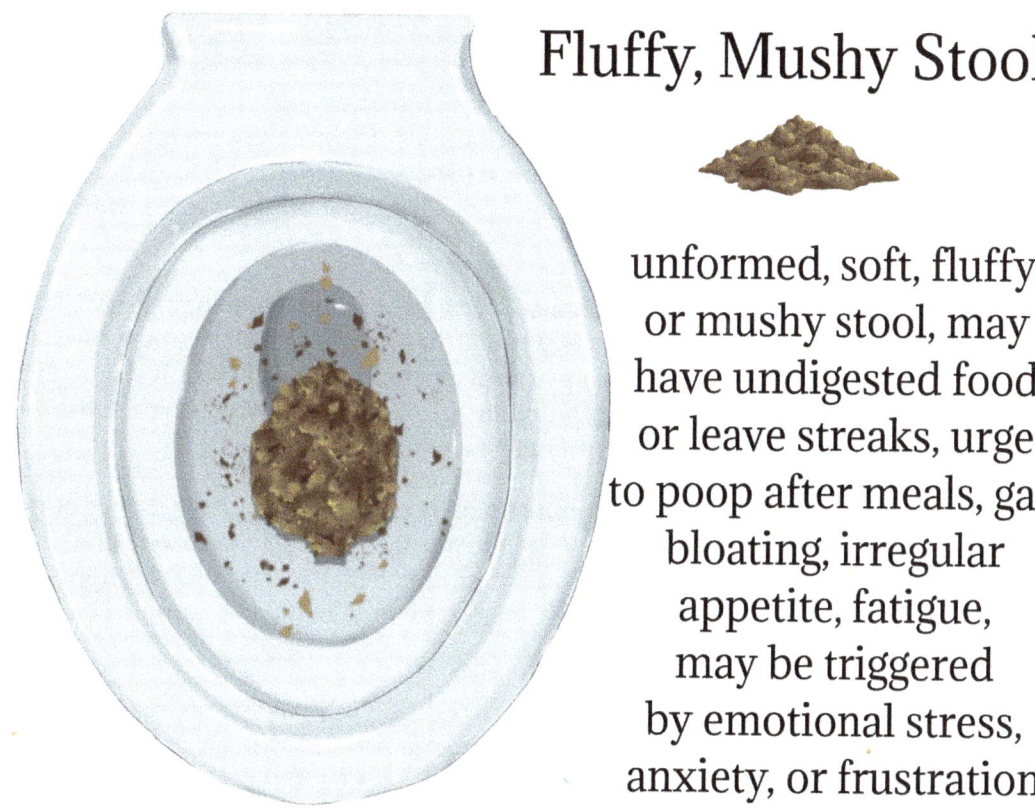

Fluffy, Mushy Stool

unformed, soft, fluffy, or mushy stool, may have undigested food or leave streaks, urge to poop after meals, gas, bloating, irregular appetite, fatigue, may be triggered by emotional stress, anxiety, or frustration

Figure 6.5 Fluffy, mushy, loose stool, Liver and Spleen disharmony.

What It Means: Fluffy pieces of stool indicate a TCM pattern of Liver Qi Attacking the Spleen. This pattern reflects an imbalance between the energies of the Liver and the Spleen. In TCM, the Liver's role is to ensure the smooth flow of Qi, including emotional and digestive flow. When Liver Qi becomes stagnant — often due to stress, frustration, or repressed emotions — it can attack the Spleen, which is responsible for digestion and nutrient absorption. This imbalance weakens the Spleen's ability to transform and transport food and fluids, resulting in loose, unformed stools.

Liver attacking the Spleen may sound strange, but it's not so different from a familiar human experience: You have a stressful day — your boss criticizes you or a meeting goes badly. You come home still frustrated and, without meaning to, take it out on your spouse or child. They feel hurt and withdraw. They weren't the cause, but they felt the impact.

Our organs, in Chinese medicine, have relationships like we do. When one is overwhelmed — like the Liver under stress — it can "attack" another, like the Spleen, disrupting balance. It's not literal violence, but a metaphor for how internal disharmony shows up — just like emotional stress affects our relationships.

When you are carefree and relaxed, Liver Qi flows smoothly. Emotions like anger or resentment agitates the Liver Qi which then disrupts the functions of the Spleen. More specifically, the Liver's energy constrains the Spleen's ability to digest and transform food into Qi and Blood. This is why you may not have much of an appetite when you are angry or you might have the sensation of food being stuck in your stomach when you do try to eat.

Underlying Causes

In Traditional Chinese Medicine, the pattern of Liver Qi attacking the Spleen describes a disharmony where the Liver's Qi becomes unbalanced and disrupts the digestive functions of the Spleen. This intricate relationship means a problem in one area can quickly ripple to another area.

Often, the primary drivers of this pattern are emotional factors, particularly chronic or intense feelings like frustration, anger, and resentment. These powerful emotions can cause the Liver's energy to become aggressive, leading it to "attack" and disrupt the Spleen's ability to process food and nutrients. Stress, whether it's from work, relationships, or life's myriad events, only exacerbates this Liver Qi stagnation. Prolonged or excessive stress can lock you into a chronic cycle of disharmony.

Your diet and habits also play a significant role. Irregular eating habits, such as skipping meals or inconsistent mealtimes, can weaken the Spleen's inherent digestive power. Furthermore, diets rich in greasy, spicy, and processed foods overburden the digestive system, creating an environment ripe for both Liver Qi stagnation and Spleen dysfunction. A sedentary lifestyle only makes things worse; regular physical activity is crucial for promoting the smooth flow of Qi throughout the body, helping to prevent stagnation.

Beyond these common causes, other factors can contribute to this pattern. Some individuals may be more susceptible to Liver Qi stagnation due to environmental or lifestyle influences. For example, a person raised in a high-strung or emotionally repressed family environment may grow up with a tendency to suppress emotions like frustration or sadness. Over time, this emotional pattern can become ingrained and manifest as chronic Liver Qi stagnation, especially under stress.

Exposure to environmental toxins and pollution can also disrupt the body's energy systems, potentially impacting both the Liver and Spleen. Lastly, hormonal imbalances — particularly in women during key phases such as puberty, menstruation, and menopause — can directly influence Liver Qi, often leading to symptoms like mood swings, breast tenderness, digestive upset, or fatigue.

Why The Liver And Spleen Need To Be In Harmony In Our Body

In Traditional Chinese Medicine, the Liver and Spleen are far more than just individual organs; they form a dynamic partnership that plays a central role in maintaining internal harmony. When these two systems function smoothly and in balance, they support the smooth flow of Qi, proper digestion, emotional stability, and the overall health of the body.

The Liver acts as the body's chief of staff, ensuring the smooth flow of Qi everywhere. When this energy flows freely, it supports everything from healthy digestion and robust circulation to stable emotions. Meanwhile, the Spleen is your body's master transformer, taking the food you eat and converting it into precious Qi and Blood. When the Liver and Spleen are in sync, Qi is readily available, powering all your bodily functions. This harmonious duo is also essential for emotional health. A balanced Liver Qi helps regulate feelings like anger, frustration, and irritability, while the Spleen's ability to nourish Blood and Qi provides a stable foundation for emotional resilience.

Beyond energy and emotions, the Liver and Spleen are the cornerstones of healthy digestion in Traditional Chinese Medicine. The Spleen is responsible for transforming food into Qi and Blood and transporting this nourishment throughout the body, while the Liver ensures the smooth flow of Qi in the digestive tract. When these two organs function in harmony, digestion becomes efficient and symptoms like bloating, indigestion, and irregular bowel movements are minimized. The Liver also plays a key role in detoxification by regulating the free flow of Qi, which supports the body's ability to process and eliminate toxins. Its balanced relationship with the Spleen helps reduce the buildup of Dampness and relieves strain on other organ systems.

Their teamwork extends to your very lifeblood and physical strength. The Liver stores and regulates Blood volume, while the Spleen is intricately involved in Blood production. This ensures your body has an adequate supply of nourishing Blood, vital for every cell and organ. Furthermore, the Liver is linked to the health of tendons and ligaments, while the Spleen nourishes your muscles. When both organs are in harmony, they contribute significantly to your overall musculoskeletal strength and flexibility.

Ultimately, disharmony between the Liver and Spleen can lead to significant issues like Qi Stagnation, Blood Stasis, and emotional imbalances. These can manifest as a wide array of health problems, including chronic digestive disorders, menstrual irregularities, persistent emotional disturbances, and musculoskeletal issues. Maintaining the balance between your Liver and Spleen is truly fundamental to your holistic well-being in TCM.

Different Individuals May Experience Different Symptoms With Fluffy Stool Pieces that are Sticky, Mushy, Loose or Soft With Or Without Undigested Food

Abdominal Pain. Individuals may experience abdominal discomfort or pain, often with a distending or bloating sensation in the upper abdomen and worsened by emotional stress.

Digestive Issues. This pattern can lead to digestive problems such as diarrhea, loose stools, or alternating between diarrhea and constipation. Emotional disturbances, stress, or frustration can trigger diarrhea. This diarrhea is typically watery and may be accompanied by urgency and frequent bowel movements. Abdominal discomfort is often relieved after a bowel movement.

Emotional Disturbances. Liver and Spleen disharmony often affects emotions. Symptoms can include irritability, mood swings, frustration, or feeling easily stressed or emotional instability.

Fatigue. People with this pattern may experience fatigue and a lack of energy, which can be related to both physical and emotional imbalances.

Appetite Changes. It can affect appetite, leading to either increased or decreased hunger. Some individuals may have cravings for certain foods.

Belching. Excessive belching or burping may occur, sometimes accompanied by a sensation of fullness or bloating in the upper abdomen.

Fullness in the Chest and Side of the Ribs. Some individuals may feel fullness or discomfort in the chest area and along side of the ribs.

Taste Changes. People may notice changes in taste, such as a bitter or sour taste in the mouth.

Loss of Appetite. Individuals with this pattern may experience a reduced appetite, especially during or after emotional episodes.

Acid Regurgitation. Acid regurgitation or acid reflux can occur, leading to a sour or bitter taste in the mouth.

Sleep Disturbances. Difficulty falling asleep or staying asleep can be associated with this pattern.

Menstrual Irregularities. For women, it can lead to irregular menstrual cycles or other gynecological issues.

Sallow Complexion. The complexion may appear sallow or dull, reflecting the disharmony between the Liver and Spleen.

Tongue. In this pattern, the tongue may show signs of white or yellow coating with areas of pale discoloration.

Self-Care and Support

Manage Stress. Since emotional factors play a significant role in Liver and Spleen disharmony, stress reduction techniques can be beneficial. These may include meditation, deep breathing exercises, yoga, or mindfulness practices.

Exercise Regularly. Engaging in regular physical activity helps promote the smooth flow of Qi and Blood in the body. Activities like walking, tai chi, or Qigong can be particularly helpful.

Modify Diet. TCM dietary principles emphasize the importance of a balanced diet. Consider the following dietary adjustments:

1. **Eat in moderation.** Avoid overeating and aim for regular, moderate meals. Irregular eating patterns can disrupt the Spleen's function.

2. **Avoid raw or cold foods.** Cold and raw foods can weaken the Spleen's digestive capacity. Opt for warm, cooked foods instead.

3. **Limit greasy foods and spicy foods.** These can exacerbate Liver Qi stagnation. Reduce or eliminate fried and heavily spiced dishes.

4. **Include foods that soothe Liver Qi.** Leafy greens, bitter melon, and foods high in fiber can help soothe Liver Qi stagnation.

Stay Hydrated. Drink plenty of water throughout the day to support overall digestive health.

Herbal Support. Bupleurum (Chai Hu), White Peony Root (Bai Shao), and Chen Pi (Tangerine Peel) to soothe Liver Qi, harmonize Spleen, and reduce Dampness.

Receive Acupuncture. Acupuncture sessions with a trained practitioner can help regulate Qi flow and address specific symptoms associated with Liver and Spleen disharmony.

Get Deep Sleep. Establish a regular sleep routine to ensure adequate rest. Sleep is crucial for overall health and emotional balance.

Foods To Relieve Disharmony Between The Liver And Spleen

Leafy green vegetables like kale, spinach, and collard greens are high in fiber and can help soothe Liver Qi stagnation.

Bitter foods can help drain excess Liver energy. Examples include bitter melon, arugula, and dandelion greens.

Cooling foods can help counteract Liver heat. Cucumber, watermelon, and mint are good choices.

Whole grains like brown rice, quinoa, and oats are nourishing for the Spleen and provide sustained energy.

Root vegetables like sweet potatoes, carrots, and beets are grounding and supportive of Spleen function.

Lean proteins, poultry, fish, and tofu provide protein necessary for overall health and energy.

Cooked foods are easier to digest than raw foods. In TCM, it's generally advised to consume warm, cooked foods rather than raw or cold foods, which can weaken the Spleen.

Legumes, like beans, lentils, and chickpeas, are a good source of protein and fiber, supporting both organs.

Apples are considered a balancing fruit in TCM and can help regulate digestion.

Chamomile tea is calming and can help soothe Liver Qi. It's a good choice if you're experiencing stress.

Ginger is warming and can help with digestion. It's often used to alleviate symptoms of Spleen deficiency.

Mint tea or fresh mint leaves can help soothe the Liver and reduce heat.

Pumpkin seeds and sunflower seeds provide essential nutrients and can be beneficial.

Green tea is packed with antioxidants and can help balance the body's energy.

Mushrooms, like shiitake and maitake, have immune-boosting properties. In TCM, mushrooms boost the Qi and nourish the Spleen.

Herbs, are soothing to the Liver, strengthen the Spleen, and harmonize digestion include Bupleurum Root (Chai Hu), White Peony Root (Bai Shao), Poria (Fu Ling), and Licorice Root (Gan Cao). It is best to work with a qualified TCM practitioner when using herbal formulas. For daily support, a balancing tea with rose buds and peppermint can help calm emotions and ease digestion.

Foods That Can Worsen Disharmony Between The Liver And Spleen

Spicy foods. Spices such as chili peppers, garlic, and onions can stimulate the Liver and create heat, making the condition worse.

Greasy and fried foods. Excessively oily and fried foods can overwhelm the Spleen's digestive capacity and lead to dampness and heat in the Liver.

Alcohol. Excessive alcohol consumption can disrupt Liver function and lead to excess heat in the Liver.

Coffee and caffeine. Caffeine-containing beverages like coffee can stimulate the Liver and contribute to Liver Qi stagnation.

Processed foods. Highly processed and artificial foods are typically difficult to digest and may disrupt Spleen function.

Excessive sugar. High-sugar diets can create dampness in the body, which can exacerbate Spleen issues.

Cold foods and drinks. Extremely cold or iced foods and drinks can weaken the Spleen's digestive fire, leading to poor digestion and dampness.

Excessively sour foods. Sour foods can contribute to Liver stagnation. This includes excessive consumption of citrus fruits and vinegar.

Red meat. While small amounts of lean red meat can be beneficial, excessive consumption can create heat in the Liver.

Dairy. Dairy products, especially in excess, can create dampness in the body and disturb Spleen function.

Excessively salty foods. Excessive salt intake can contribute to dampness and affect Spleen function.

Raw foods. In TCM, raw foods are generally considered more challenging to digest, so they may not be ideal for individuals with Spleen issues.

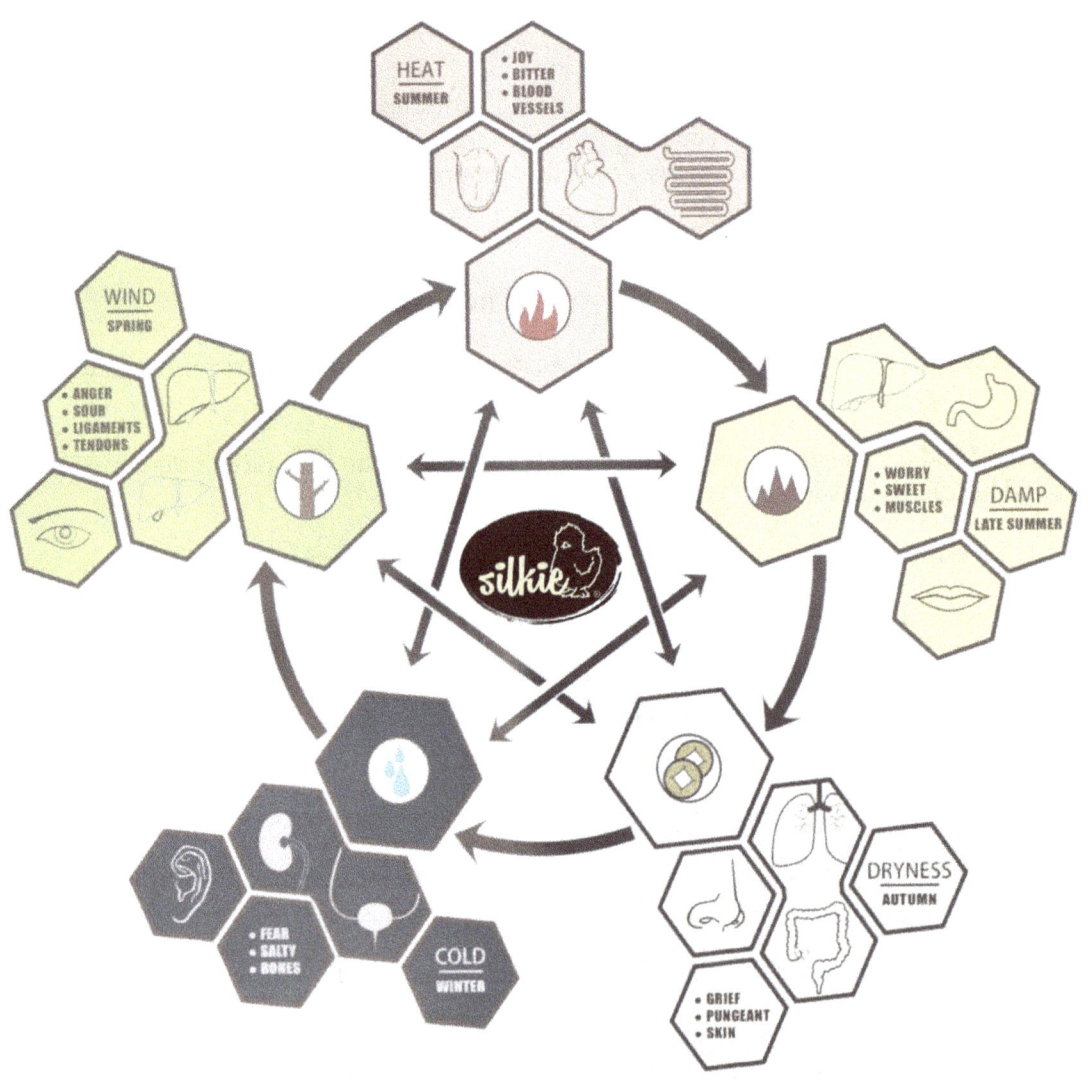

6. Stool With White Dots or Thin White Worms - Sign of parasite

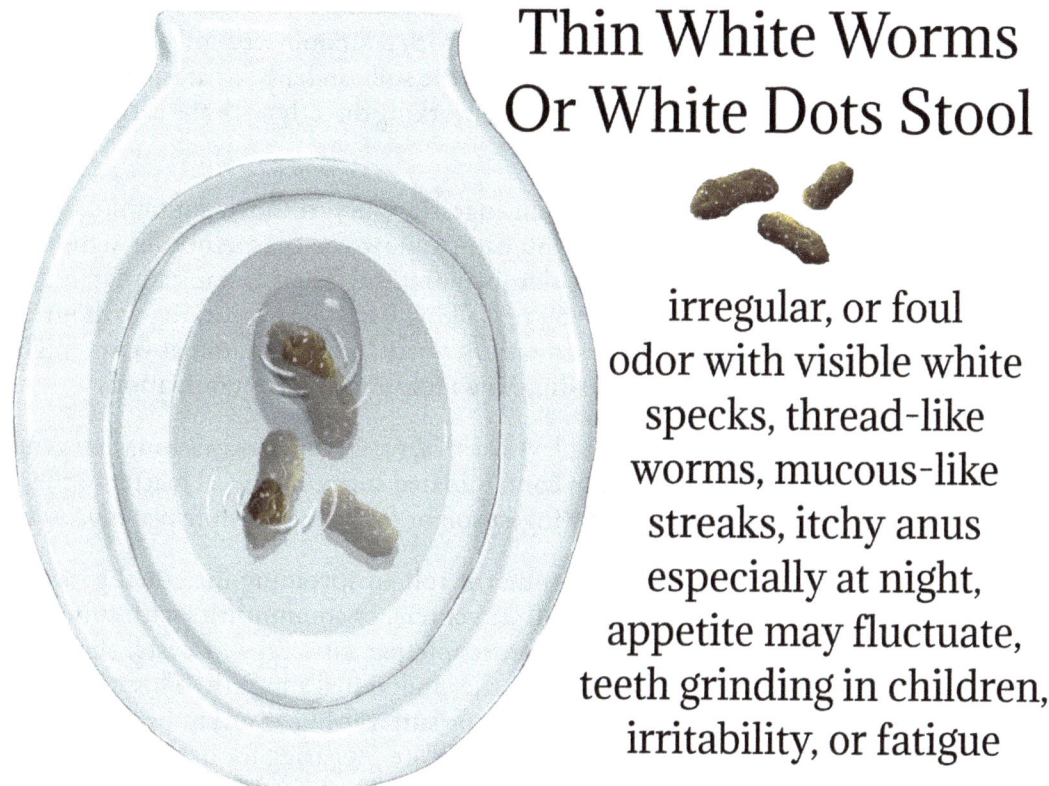

Thin White Worms Or White Dots Stool

irregular, or foul odor with visible white specks, thread-like worms, mucous-like streaks, itchy anus especially at night, appetite may fluctuate, teeth grinding in children, irritability, or fatigue

Figure 6.6 White dots or thin white worms in stool, Intestinal Parasites or Weak Spleen Function.

What It Means: Soft stool containing white dots or thin white worms, accompanied by long-term abdominal pain and morning diarrhea. In Traditional Chinese Medicine, this points to Spleen Qi Deficiency allowing parasites or Dampness in the Intestines. The Spleen, responsible for transforming and transporting food and nutrients, also plays a vital role in keeping the digestive tract clean and protected. When the Spleen is weak — due to poor diet, overconsumption of cold/raw food or raw fish, like sushi or sashimi, excessive sugar, or chronic stress — it loses its ability to control Dampness and defend against pathogenic organisms.

Parasites are considered a form of internal Damp-Heat or Toxicity in TCM. Parasites often thrive in individuals with weakened digestive fire and poor immunity. Children are especially susceptible due to their still-developing Spleen. Despite modern advancements in sanitation, parasitic infections remain common and can be transmitted through contaminated food, water, or contact with infected animals.

Various parasites can affect the digestive system, with Anisakis and Spirometra being two of the most frequently encountered. Anisakis, a type of nematode (roundworm), can cause acute symptoms such as abdominal pain, nausea, vomiting, diarrhea, hematemesis (vomiting blood), and sometimes urticaria (hives), depending on the site of invasion within the body. In contrast, Spirometra, a type of tapeworm, generally produces milder effects than roundworm infections, with symptoms that are subtle and often go unnoticed for long periods.

Underlying Causes

Parasitic infections, particularly those affecting the intestines, often stem from a range of environmental and behavioral factors. Understanding these underlying causes is key to preventing their spread.

One of the most common culprits is consuming contaminated water and food. This happens when water sources or food items are tainted with parasitic cysts, eggs, or larvae. Such contamination is particularly prevalent in areas with inadequate sanitation and poor hygiene infrastructure. Similarly, eating undercooked or raw meat from infected animals, like pork or beef, can directly transmit certain parasites, such as tapeworms.

For those who enjoy gardening or agricultural work, contact with contaminated soil can also lead to infection with specific soil-transmitted parasites. This occurs because the soil can harbor parasitic eggs or larvae, often from the feces of infected humans or animals. When you're working directly with the earth, these microscopic organisms can find their way into your body.

One common way this happens is through inadvertent ingestion: if you touch contaminated soil and then touch your mouth without proper handwashing, you can swallow the eggs. Another significant route for some parasites, like hookworms, is through direct skin penetration. Their larvae can hatch in the soil and then actively burrow into your skin, especially if you're walking barefoot or working without gloves. These infections are more prevalent in areas with poor sanitation where human or animal waste might be used as fertilizer or where open defecation is practiced, leading to widespread soil contamination.

Beyond environmental exposure, personal hygiene plays a critical role. Poor handwashing and general personal hygiene can easily transfer parasitic organisms from contaminated surfaces or fecal matter to the mouth. This risk is amplified in children who may inadvertently ingest soil or fecal matter while playing.

Direct human-to-human contact can also play a significant role in spreading intestinal parasites, especially within close-knit environments like households, childcare centers, or communities with suboptimal hygiene. This often occurs via the fecal-oral route, where microscopic parasitic eggs or cysts, shed in the stool of an infected person, are inadvertently transferred to another individual's mouth. This can happen through contaminated hands, shared objects like toys or utensils, or surfaces like doorknobs or bathroom fixtures. The lack of thorough handwashing after using the toilet or before preparing food creates an easy pathway for these resilient parasites to spread, turning a single infection into a cluster of cases within a family or a wider community.

Travel also poses a significant risk; visiting regions where intestinal parasites are endemic naturally increases the likelihood of exposure to contaminated food and water. On a broader scale, inadequate sanitation, specifically a lack of access to clean toilet facilities, is a major contributor to the widespread transmission of these parasites. Equally important is inadequate health education. A lack of awareness about proper hygiene and sanitation practices directly correlates with a higher risk of parasitic infections. Finally, individuals with a weakened immune system, such as those living with HIV/AIDS or undergoing immunosuppressive therapy, are often more susceptible to contracting and experiencing severe symptoms from intestinal parasitic infections.

How Intestinal Parasitic Infection Can Affect Our Body

Intestinal parasitic infections can significantly impact your body's well-being, leading to a range of symptoms, including unintended weight loss. Here's how these microscopic invaders can wreak havoc:

Parasites primarily target your digestive system, acting like unwelcome guests that disrupt its normal functioning. They can lead to diarrhea, abdominal pain, bloating, and irregular bowel movements. This is because parasites can weaken the vital functions of your Spleen and Stomach, which are crucial for proper digestion. When these organs are out of sync, your body struggles to break down food and absorb essential nutrients. This malabsorption can directly contribute to unintended weight loss as your body isn't getting the nourishment it needs, even if you're eating regularly.

Chronic parasitic infections can deplete your body's Qi and Blood, leaving you feeling exhausted and weak. This deficiency often manifests as fatigue, a pale complexion, and a general lack of vitality. When your Qi and Blood are low, every bodily function can suffer, including your ability to maintain a healthy weight.

Some parasitic infections can lead to an accumulation of dampness and phlegm in the body. This can result in uncomfortable symptoms like mucous or greasy stools, a heavy sensation in your body, and even cognitive fog. Additionally, certain parasites can create an environment where heat and toxins build up. When these levels surpass a healthy threshold, you might experience symptoms like fever and skin issues.

Parasitic infections can disrupt the smooth flow of Blood and Qi, leading to stagnation. This can cause symptoms such as abdominal pain, headaches, and general discomfort. Furthermore, chronic parasitic infections can weaken your Wei Qi, which is your body's protective energy, similar to your immune system. A compromised Wei Qi makes you more vulnerable to recurrent illnesses, further taxing your body's resources.

The impact of parasitic infections isn't limited to the physical. Prolonged infections can also significantly affect your emotional and psychological well-being. Parasites absorb nutrients, reducing the availability of Qi and Blood needed to support emotional and mental stability. This deficiency can lead to feelings of irritability, anxiety, and restlessness.

Understanding how these infections impact your body is the first step toward seeking appropriate treatment and restoring your health.

Different Individuals May Experience Different Symptoms With Stool containing White Dots or Thin White Worms

Gastrointestinal Symptoms. Diarrhea, constipation, abdominal pain or cramps, bloating, gas, nausea, vomiting, and loss of appetite are common symptoms.

Stool Changes. Bowel movements may become more frequent and stools may change in color, consistency, and odor. Additionally there can be blood or mucus in the stool.

Fatigue and Weakness. Chronic parasite infections can lead to fatigue and a general sense of weakness because parasites steal nutrients and weaken digestion, leaving the body undernourished. In TCM, this is seen as Damp-Heat damaging the Spleen and leading to Qi and Blood deficiency.

Weight Loss: Persistent infections can cause unintended weight loss.

Skin Issues. Rash or itching, especially around the anus (may indicate pinworms), and hives can be common with parasitic infections.

Anal and Rectal Symptoms. There may be itching, irritation, pain, or discomfort in the area.

Nutritional Deficiencies. Some parasites can interfere with nutrient absorption, leading to deficiencies in vitamins and minerals. This can result in symptoms like anemia.

Sleep Disturbances. Certain parasitic infections, such as pinworms, can lead to disturbed sleep due to itching and discomfort, especially at night.

Cognitive and Emotional Symptoms. Difficulty concentrating may be more common in children. Irritability, anxiety, and restlessness can arise.

Fever. In some cases, parasitic infections can cause a low-grade fever.

Allergic Reactions. Some individuals may experience allergic reactions, such as hives or swelling, in response to parasitic infections.

Respiratory Symptoms. In rare cases, parasitic larvae can migrate to the Lungs, leading to symptoms like coughing and wheezing.

Self-Care and Support

Hygiene and Sanitation:

1. Practice good hand hygiene by washing your hands thoroughly with soap and clean water after using the toilet, before eating, and after handling soil or contaminated objects.

2. Maintain clean and sanitary living conditions, including regular cleaning of bathroom facilities.

3. To reduce the risk of parasitic infections, avoid consuming contaminated water — especially when traveling to high-risk areas. Always opt for boiled or properly filtered water.

4. Wash fruits and vegetables thoroughly before eating or cooking them.

Food Safety:

1. Ensure that food is cooked thoroughly, especially meat and seafood, to kill any potential parasites.

2. Avoid consuming undercooked or raw meat, fish, or shellfish.

3. Be cautious when eating in areas with poor food hygiene practices.

Personal Hygiene:

1. Keep fingernails trimmed and clean to reduce the risk of transferring parasites from contaminated surfaces to your mouth.

2. Teach children the importance of proper handwashing and hygiene practices.

Avoiding Soil Contamination:

1. Wear shoes and avoid walking barefoot, especially in areas where soil may be contaminated with parasites.

2. If you handle soil or work in a garden, wear gloves and wash your hands thoroughly afterward.

Travel Precautions:

1. When traveling to regions where parasitic infections are more common, take precautions to avoid consuming contaminated water and food.

2. Consider consulting a travel medicine specialist for advice on specific travel-related risks.

Community Education: In areas with a high prevalence of parasitic infections, community education programs can help raise awareness about prevention and hygiene practices.

Follow-Up Testing: After completing the prescribed treatment for a parasitic infection, follow up with your healthcare provider for additional testing to ensure that the infection has been successfully treated and that there are no lingering parasites.

Supportive Care: Depending on the severity of symptoms, your healthcare provider may recommend supportive care, such as rehydration therapy, to manage symptoms like diarrhea and dehydration.

Prevent Re-Infection: Take steps to prevent re-infection by continuing to practice good hygiene and food safety measures even after treatment.

Foods To Relieve Intestinal Parasitic Infection

Garlic is known for its potential antimicrobial properties and may help combat some parasites. It can be added to cooked dishes or taken as a supplement under medical supervision.

Pumpkin seeds may have anti-parasitic properties. They can be eaten raw, roasted, or ground into a paste and added to foods.

Ginger has anti-inflammatory and immune-boosting properties and can be included in teas or meals to support digestive health.

Probiotic-rich foods such as sauerkraut, kimchi, and other fermented vegetables contain beneficial bacteria that can support gut health during and after a parasitic infection. Yogurt also contains probiotics, but as a dairy product that is cold in nature, it may weaken the Spleen and promote Dampness.

High-fiber foods, including whole grains, fruits, and vegetables, can help regulate bowel movements and ease digestive discomfort.

Hydration is crucial during and after parasitic infections, as diarrhea and vomiting can lead to dehydration. Drink plenty of clean, purified water to stay hydrated.

Herbs to expel parasites, strengthen digestion, and stop discomfort include Smoked Plum (Wu Mei), Chinaberry Tree Bark (Ku Lian Pi), and Areca Seed (Bing Lang). It is best to work with a qualified TCM practitioner when using herbal formulas. For daily support, herbal teas with wormwood (Qing Hao) and pomegranate peel can support parasite-clearing regimens.

Fruits and vegetables provide essential vitamins and minerals that support the body's immune system. Opt for a variety of colorful fruits and vegetables to ensure a diverse range of nutrients.

Lean proteins, such as poultry, fish, tofu, and legumes, can help support the body's immune system and overall recovery.

Follow medical advice. Always follow the prescribed treatment plan provided by your healthcare provider. Medications are typically the primary means of treating parasitic infections.

Maintain food safety to prevent re-infection. Ensure that all foods are cooked thoroughly, especially meat and seafood. Practice good food hygiene and wash hands before handling food.

Foods That Can Worsen Intestinal Parasitic Infection

Sugary and processed foods tend to have artificial additives and preservatives and can weaken the immune system and promote inflammation, potentially making the body more vulnerable to parasitic infections. Avoid or limit sugary snacks, candies, and processed foods.

Dairy consumption can create dampness in the body, which may provide a favorable environment for parasites. Consider moderating your intake of dairy products.

Raw or undercooked meat and seafood can increase the risk of parasitic infections. Ensure that meat and seafood are cooked thoroughly to kill any potential parasites.

Contaminated water and unwashed produce can also cause parasitic infections. Be cautious about the source of your water, and wash fresh produce thoroughly before consumption.

Excessively cold or raw foods weaken the digestive system and may create an environment that is more susceptible to parasites. Balance your diet with cooked and warm foods, especially if you suspect a parasitic infection.

Alcohol and caffeine can dehydrate the body and weaken the immune system. Consider reducing or avoiding alcohol and caffeinated beverages during recovery.

Greasy and fried foods can cause stagnation (indigestion) which can exacerbate digestive issues and may not be conducive to healing.

Overeating can strain the digestive system, potentially making it easier for parasites to thrive. Practice portion control and avoid overeating.

Laxative abuse can disrupt the natural balance of the digestive system, potentially contributing to digestive issues. Avoid excessive use of laxatives.

Processed meats, such as sausages and hot dogs, may contain additives and preservatives that could potentially weaken the immune system. Limit processed meat consumption.

7. Soft Blobs That Require Some Straining To Pass - Indicative of initial onset of Qi and Blood Deficiency

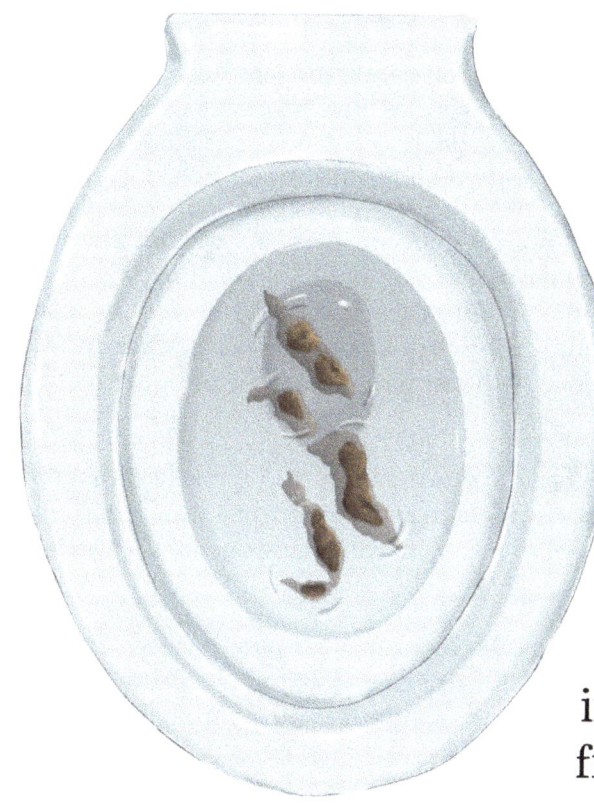

Soft Blobs Of Stool

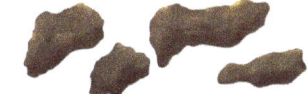

lacks solid form, may appear as soft clumps or scattered blobs, may float or be difficult to flush, incomplete evacuation, frequent urges, bloating

Figure 6.7 Soft blobs of poop, early stage of Blood and Qi deficiency, Spleen Qi Deficiency or Dampness in the Intestines.

What It Means: If you have to strain to pass soft blobs of poop, then this is an indication of Qi and Blood Deficiency. Soft stools are due to digestive weakness, more specifically a Spleen deficiency pattern in TCM. Digestive weakness means food cannot be fully digested and converted into energy and Blood for the body to use. Overtime, impaired digestive function naturally leads to a decline in Qi and Blood production. Having to strain means there is not enough energy or Qi for peristalsis to push the stool out.

Underlying Causes

Ever wonder why you might feel perpetually drained or look a little lackluster? In the holistic view of Traditional Chinese Medicine, these signs often point to a deficiency of Blood and Qi, the dynamic duo that fuels and nourishes our entire being. Let's delve into the common culprits that can leave these vital substances running low.

Think of your digestive system as a hardworking kitchen that never stops, constantly turning food into the essential energy (Qi) and nourishment (Blood) your body depends on. If you're not eating well – skipping meals or relying on low-quality foods – it's like trying to cook a meal with an empty fridge and missing ingredients. Without the right fuel, your body can't make enough Qi and Blood to keep you feeling strong and vibrant.

Regularly missing meals, avoiding nutrient-rich foods, or overloading on cold and raw items – like endless salads and smoothies – can weaken your digestive fire and slow the body's ability to create Qi and Blood. In TCM, warm, cooked foods are preferred because they're easier to digest and absorb, allowing your inner "kitchen" to work more efficiently.

Then there are the persistent challenges of prolonged or chronic illnesses. Imagine your body constantly battling an unseen foe. This ongoing struggle consumes precious resources, and in TCM terms, many chronic conditions involve inflammation, which acts like a roadblock, blocking the creation and smooth flow of Qi and Blood. Inflammation in the Lungs, for example, makes it harder to breathe deeply and limits oxygen intake. With less oxygen, your organs can't function optimally to generate and circulate vital Qi and Blood. It's a cumulative effect, where long-term illness steadily drains our reserves and leaves us depleted.

Our bodies are designed to conserve, so losing too much Blood can significantly impact our energy levels. Excessive Blood loss, whether from heavy menstrual cycles, injuries, surgery, or even frequent nosebleeds, directly depletes this vital substance. Women experiencing heavy periods are particularly vulnerable, as Blood is what nourishes our muscles, organs, and, well, everything! Losing too much is like draining the fuel tank.

The invisible weight of our emotions can also take a heavy toll. Chronic stress, anxiety, and emotional turmoil act like a constant drain on our energy reserves, disrupting the natural flow of Qi. Think of stress as putting your body into a perpetual "fight or flight" mode. While helpful in short bursts, this state burns through a lot of energy. Staying in this high-alert mode for too long leads to exhaustion, a clear sign of Blood and Qi deficiency. In TCM, emotional balance isn't just a mental state; it's deeply intertwined with our physical health, and unresolved emotions can significantly impact our vital energies.

Even our well-intentioned efforts can sometimes backfire. Physical overexertion, especially without proper rest and recovery, can deplete our Qi and Blood stores. In our busy modern lives, this might look like pushing ourselves too hard at the gym, working relentlessly for long hours, or engaging in demanding mental or physical tasks without giving our bodies a chance to replenish.

The importance of good sleep cannot be overstated in TCM. Inadequate or poor-quality sleep directly weakens our Qi and Blood reserves. Think of sleep as the body's nightly recharge. If we're awake during the hours when our bodies naturally want to rest and rebuild, our brains and bodies continue to burn through precious Qi and Blood without proper replenishment.

The passage of time itself plays a role. Aging is a natural process that leads to a gradual decline in our ability to produce and replenish vital substances like Qi and Blood. It's a natural ebb and flow – a vibrant teenager typically has more energy than someone in their thirties, who in turn will generally have more than someone in their seventies.

Sometimes, our starting point influences our resilience. Some individuals have a constitutional predisposition to Qi and Blood Deficiency, making them more susceptible from birth. For example, babies born prematurely may naturally have lower initial reserves.

Our external environment can also be a drain. Exposure to harsh conditions, like extreme cold or dampness, forces our bodies to expend extra energy. In a bitter cold climate, we burn more calories (energy) just to stay warm. In persistently humid or rainy weather, the body can feel heavy and sluggish, requiring more effort for even simple tasks, thus depleting our Qi.

Finally, a compromised digestive system can create a vicious cycle. Chronic digestive issues, such as malabsorption, GERD, ulcers, SIBO, Crohn's, or IBS, impair our ability to properly extract nutrients from food. If our "kitchen" isn't working efficiently, we can't produce enough Qi and Blood, no matter how well we eat. Interestingly, in TCM, persistent digestive issues can sometimes manifest as thinness (due to lack of nourishment) or a disproportionately large belly (due to undigested food turning into dampness or mucus). It's all interconnected in the fascinating web of Traditional Chinese Medicine!

The Importance of Blood and Qi

In the vibrant language of Traditional Chinese Medicine, the concepts of Blood and Qi are like the inseparable Yin and Yang, the very foundation upon which our health is built. Think of Blood not just as the familiar red fluid coursing through your veins, delivering life-giving oxygen and nutrients to every cell, but as something even more encompassing. Blood is the rich, nourishing essence that moistens our tissues, warms our limbs, and carries vital substances throughout our being.

The Blood within your body is much like the Earth beneath your feet, providing the very foundation for all life. Earth is rich in minerals and nutrients, the essential ingredients that allow plants to grow and animals to thrive. Similarly, Blood within our bodies is the fertile ground that nourishes every single cell, tissue, and organ. It carries the "minerals" of our food – the essential nutrients – and the "water" of life-giving oxygen, allowing our internal "ecosystem" to flourish.

Think about how the Earth provides moisture, preventing dryness and allowing for flexibility and growth. Blood does the same within us, keeping our skin supple, our joints lubricated, and our internal organs functioning smoothly. Just as a parched land withers, insufficient Blood leads to dryness and a lack of vitality throughout the body.

Furthermore, the Earth has a natural warmth, radiating from its core and warmed by the sun. This warmth sustains life and allows for all the dynamic processes of nature. Similarly, Blood carries a warming quality, maintaining our body temperature and ensuring that all our tissues are vital and active. When Blood is deficient, we might feel cold easily, a sign of insufficient internal warmth.

Finally, the Earth stores and transports vital resources. Rivers carry water to nourish the land, and the soil holds the nutrients that plants need. In the same way, Blood acts as our internal river system, transporting nutrients, hormones, and other essential substances to where they are needed, ensuring the smooth functioning and communication between all parts of our "internal landscape."

So, when we think of Blood as the Earth, we're not just talking about a red fluid. We're envisioning the fundamental, grounding, nourishing, moisturizing, and warming substance that provides the very basis for life within us, much like the Earth does for the world around us. It's the rich soil from which our vitality springs.

Interestingly, even our sweat is considered an extension of this precious Blood. A healthy glow after exercise? That's Blood doing its job! But excessive sweating, whether from pushing yourself too hard or those unsettling night sweats, can actually deplete this vital substance, leaving us feeling drained.

Now, meet Qi, often translated as "energy," but it's more like the dynamic force that animates everything. If Blood is the Earth, then Qi is the Sun, the vital energy that makes life possible. It's the power that propels the Blood, ensuring those essential nutrients reach every corner of our body. In TCM wisdom, there's a beautiful interplay: "Blood is the mother of Qi, and Qi is the commander of the Blood." This means that while Blood provides the fundamental nourishment for all our bodily functions, it can't do its job without the active, driving force of Qi to circulate it effectively. They are two sides of the same coin, working in harmony to keep our inner world vibrant and balanced. Without sufficient Blood, our bodies lack the essential building blocks; without sufficient Qi, those building blocks can't get where they need to go to keep everything running smoothly.

Qi also animates our physiology, governing how our organs function. Think of Qi as having a natural directionality: it can move upwards, downwards, inwards, and outwards. Take digestion, for instance. When you eat, the chewed food naturally travels downwards from the Stomach to the Intestines – that's the Stomach's Qi flowing in its proper direction. But when you're nauseous and vomiting, the Stomach Qi rebels, moving upwards against its natural flow. In TCM, remedies like specific herbs or acupuncture points are often used to gently guide that rebellious Stomach Qi back downwards, restoring harmony.

Ultimately, Qi is the driving force behind all our bodily functions – from the intricate dance of digestion and circulation to the simple act of movement and the vigilant shield of our immunity. It's the umbrella term encompassing all the different types of "energy" that bring life to our physical form. Think of mechanical energy for our muscles to move, electrical energy powering our heartbeat and nerve impulses for sensation and thought, and biochemical energy fueling the tireless work within our cells. Qi encompasses all of this and more, including the subtle energies that underpin our metabolic processes, physiological functions, mental clarity, and the vibrant tapestry of our emotions. It's the very essence of being alive!

Within human physiology, TCM organizes Qi into 5 major types: Original Qi (Yuan Qi), Nutritive Qi (Ying Qi), Gathering Qi (Zong Qi), Defensive Qi (Wei Qi), and Organ Qi (Zang-Fu Qi). Each type has specific functions and locations in the body.

Original Qi, also known as Source Qi, is inherited from our parents and stored in the Kidneys. The health of our parents (mentally, physically, and emotionally) at the time of our conception determines the strength of our Source Qi and our constitution or genetics. Source Qi supports growth, development, and reproductive functions. Source Qi can only be conserved – it cannot be replenished.

Ying Qi is Nutritive or Nourishing Qi. Nutritive Qi is extracted from food and fluids by the digestive system, most notably by the Spleen. Nutritive Qi circulates in the blood vessels and nourishes the body's organs and tissues. Whereas Source Qi is prenatal (inherited) and cannot be replenished, Nutritive Qi is post-natal and can be replenished. Therefore, maintaining a strong digestive system and eating nutritious foods at appropriate times are of utmost importance.

Zong Qi is Gathering Qi or Ancestral Qi. Gathering Qi is derived from the air we breathe and the food we eat. Because air is free and food is not, we often neglect the importance of breathing. Qi cultivating exercises like "Gathering the Qi" or meditative breathwork can strengthen Gathering Qi which accumulates in the chest and supports the Lungs with respiration and the Heart with circulation. When Gathering Qi is deficient, it can manifest clinically as a weak voice, difficulty breathing, and poor circulation.

Wei Qi or Defensive Qi circulates outside the blood vessels and functions much like the immune system. The job of Defensive Qi is to protect the body from external pathogens, regulate body temperature, and control the opening and closing of skin pores. The skin is our first line of defense externally and internally we have white blood cells and antibodies to protect us from external pathogens like bacteria and viruses. Rather than a microscopic focus on bacteria and viruses, TCM takes a macroscopic view of external pathogens and ascribes a general quality like cold, heat, and damp to foreign invaders. For example, if you catch a respiratory infection and are afflicted with high fever, a rapid pulse, irritability and insatiable thirst, then your body has been overwhelmed by a heat pathogen.

Zang-Fu Qi is Organ Qi. TCM divides the organs into solid (Zang) organs and hollow (Fu) organs. Zang organs consist primarily of the Heart, Lungs, Liver, Kidneys, and Spleen which are responsible for engendering and storing Blood and Qi. Fu organs such as the Stomach, Small Intestine, Large Intestine, Gallbladder, and Bladder are hollow in nature and therefore have a greater responsibility for transporting substances like food and waste. These solid and hollow organs are all interconnected and must function harmoniously together to maintain health. Zang-Fu Qi is the vital energy for all the organs to function individually and collectively. The organs have functions that are interrelated. For example, if the Lungs break down and respiration is impaired, the Heart and other organs will be affected. Zang-Fu theory emphasizes the fact that organs do not exist nor function in isolation.

Now that you're familiar with the concepts of Blood and Qi in TCM, you can better understand why their deficiencies present with such distinct "signature symptoms." For Blood Deficiency, you'll often see fatigue, a pale complexion, dizziness, palpitations, dry skin, brittle or pale nails, and for women, scanty or irregular menstruation. When it comes to Qi Deficiency, fatigue is also common, but it's accompanied by weakness, shortness of breath, sweating with minimal exertion, poor digestion, and a tendency to get sick easily. Let's delve deeper into how these two vital energies manifest their absence in the body.

Imagine your body as a bustling metropolis and Blood as the vital delivery system, carrying precious oxygen and nutrients to every nook and cranny – from your hardworking muscles to your brilliant brain and all your essential organs. Now, what happens if this delivery system runs low? Well, you'll feel it! Fatigue sets in, like the city running out of fuel. Your head might spin and your Heart might flutter (dizziness and palpitations) because those vital supplies aren't reaching your command center and engine room effectively. Look in the mirror – a pale complexion, dry, lackluster skin, and brittle, pale nails are like distress signals from tissues and extremities that aren't getting the nourishment they crave. And for women, Blood Deficiency can throw the menstrual cycle into disarray, often leading to irregular, delayed, and scanty periods.

Now, let's talk about Qi, that incredible functional energy that animates everything we do. If your Qi levels are low, it's like the city's power grid is down. You'll feel fatigued and weak, lacking the oomph to tackle your day. Catching your breath after minimal effort (shortness of breath) and breaking a sweat easily are often whispers of weakened Lung and Heart Qi, the energy centers for respiration and circulation. A rumbling, unhappy tummy (poor digestion) often points to a sluggish Spleen Qi, the organ responsible for transforming food into usable energy. These are all examples of Zang-Fu Qi, the specific energy of our vital organs. And that annoying tendency to catch every bug that floats by? That's often a sign of a weakened Wei Qi, your body's valiant defensive force, struggling to protect the city gates!

The beauty of Traditional Chinese Medicine is its ability to see these patterns and understand the underlying imbalances. When a TCM practitioner identifies these signs of Blood or Qi deficiency, they become like skilled city planners and engineers, carefully selecting the right tools – be it the power of specific herbs, the strategic placement of acupuncture needles, or the flowing movements of Qi Gong – to revitalize the system, address the root of the deficiency, and bring your inner metropolis back into vibrant balance.

Different Individuals May Experience Different Symptoms With Soft Blobs of Stool

Abdominal Discomfort. This condition might also come with sensations of fullness in your chest and on the sides of the ribcage, frequent belching, a reduced appetite, and bloating.

Fatigue. A pervasive sense of tiredness and low energy that is not alleviated by rest.

Pale Complexion. The skin may appear pale, lacking healthy color and vitality.

Dizziness. Frequent or intermittent dizziness, especially upon standing or sudden movements.

Palpitations. Awareness of the heartbeat or a sensation of irregular heartbeats, often associated with a weak pulse.

Shortness of Breath. Breathlessness, particularly with physical exertion or even during rest.

Weakness. Generalized weakness in the muscles, making tasks and movements more challenging.

Poor Concentration. Difficulty focusing or concentrating, mental fogginess, and forgetfulness.

Pale Lips and Nails. The lips and nails may lack healthy color and appear pale.

Dry Skin and Hair. Dryness and lack of moisture in the skin and hair, potentially leading to brittle nails and hair.

Scanty Menstruation. Women may experience light or irregular menstrual periods.

Insomnia. Difficulty falling asleep or staying asleep throughout the night.

Susceptibility to illness. A weakened immune system (Defensive Qi) makes individuals more prone to frequent illnesses and infections.

Tongue. In TCM diagnosis, practitioners often examine the tongue. A pale tongue with a thin or white coating is characteristic of Blood and Qi deficiency.

Self-Care And Support

Qi Gong and Tai Chi. These gentle exercises focus on breath control, movement, and meditation, helping to cultivate Qi and enhance overall well-being.

Stress Management. Emotional stress can contribute to Qi deficiency. Practice stress reduction techniques like meditation, deep breathing exercises, or mindfulness to help manage stress.

Adequate Rest. Ensure you get enough quality sleep, as rest is crucial for replenishing Qi and Blood.

Moderate Exercise. Engage in regular, moderate exercise to boost circulation and energy levels. Avoid excessive or strenuous workouts that may further deplete your resources.

Hydration. Stay well-hydrated with water and herbal teas to support the body's functions.

Avoid Overexertion. Be mindful not to overwork yourself physically or mentally. Pace yourself and prioritize self-care.

Regular Check-Ups. If you suspect Blood and Qi deficiency, consult with a TCM practitioner for a thorough assessment and personalized treatment plan.

Emotional Balance. TCM recognizes the close connection between emotions and health. Seek emotional balance and consider practices like acupuncture, meditation, or herbal remedies that address emotional aspects.

Herbal Support. Consult with a qualified TCM practitioner who can prescribe herbal formulas tailored to your specific pattern of deficiency.

Acupuncture: Acupuncture sessions can help fortify Qi and Blood in the body, promoting balance and vitality.

Foods To Relieve Blood And Qi Deficiency

Balanced diet. Consume a balanced diet that includes a variety of foods rich in nutrients. Focus on foods that nourish Blood and Qi, such as food that is listed below.

Iron-rich foods. Lean meats, poultry, fish, and dark leafy greens.

Lean meat. Lean meats like chicken, turkey, and small amounts of lean cuts of beef are rich in iron and protein, which can help nourish Blood.

Dark leafy greens. Vegetables like spinach, kale, and Swiss chard are high in iron, folate, and vitamins, making them excellent choices for nourishing Blood.

Red dates (jujube). Red dates are a traditional remedy for Blood Deficiency. They can be added to soups, porridge, or used in herbal teas.

Goji berries. Goji berries, also known as wolfberries, are believed to tonify both Blood and Qi. They can be consumed as a snack, added to teas, or used in soups.

Black sesame seeds. Black sesame seeds are considered beneficial for nourishing Blood and are often used in TCM recipes.

Sweet potatoes. Sweet potatoes are a warming and nourishing food that can support Qi and Blood.

Brown rice. Whole grains like brown rice are a good source of complex carbohydrates and can provide sustained energy.

Beans and legumes. Beans, lentils, and chickpeas are high in protein and can help support Blood and Qi.

Tofu. While tofu is a versatile source of plant-based protein, in TCM it is considered cold in nature and may generate Dampness. For individuals with Spleen Qi Deficiency or Blood Deficiency, excessive tofu can weaken digestion and worsen fatigue, bloating, or loose stools. If included, it should be eaten sparingly, cooked with warming ingredients (such as ginger, garlic, or green onions) to balance its cold properties.

Beets. Beets are known for their Blood-nourishing properties and can be consumed as a side dish.

Molasses. Blackstrap molasses is a natural sweetener rich in iron and can be used in cooking and baking.

Nuts. Almonds, walnuts, and pine nuts are nutritious snacks that provide essential fatty acids and protein.

Ginseng. Ginseng is an adaptogenic herb to tonify Qi and promote overall vitality. It can be used in herbal teas or supplements.

Astragalus root. Astragalus is another Qi-tonifying herb often used in TCM. It can be added to soups and stews.

Ginger. Ginger is warming and a small amount can aid digestion, which is essential for Qi and Blood production.

Herbs. Herbs to tonify Qi, generate Blood, and support bowel movement include Codonopsis (Dang Shen), Angelica Root (Dang Gui), Prepared Rehmannia Root (Shu Di Huang), and White Peony Root (Bai Shao). It is best to work with a qualified TCM practitioner when using herbal formulas. For daily support, a nourishing tea of astragalus, goji berries, and jujubes can gently strengthen Qi and Blood.

Foods That Can Worsen Blood And Qi Deficiency

Cold foods and beverages hinder the Stomach and Spleen's ability to digest food, leading to poor digestion and reduced Qi and Blood production. The stomach wall is made of smooth muscle that needs to contract to churn and digest food. You would not soak your legs in cold water prior to sprinting 100 meters. Why would you drench your stomach with an ice-cold soda beverage before eating a meal? Ice-cold drinks impede your stomach's ability to digest food. Therefore, avoiding frequent or excessive consumption of ice-cold drinks, ice cream, or foods directly from the refrigerator can greatly benefit your digestion.

Raw foods are considered "cold" in TCM. Raw foods in excess are challenging for the digestive system and weaken the Spleen's function. Opt for cooked or lightly steamed vegetables and grains instead.

Dairy products like milk, cheese, and yogurt can create Dampness in the body, potentially affecting digestion and the circulation of Qi. Some individuals are more sensitive to dairy than others. In general, even those with healthy digestion may find that regular consumption of dairy weakens their system over time.

Processed and refined foods often lack essential nutrients and can contribute to Blood and Qi deficiency. These include sugary snacks, fast food, and foods high in artificial additives.

Sugary foods consumed in excess leads to fluctuations in blood sugar levels and contributes to Qi and Blood imbalances. Reducing sugar intake is beneficial.

Greasy or fried foods are difficult to digest and lead to Dampness in the body. Limiting consumption of deep-fried and greasy foods is best for those who have digestive issues, are overweight, or have oily skin.

Refrigerated or frozen foods that have been stored for extended periods. These are considered energetically cold and weaken the Spleen and Stomach with regular consumption over time.

Overeating places a burden on the digestive system, making it difficult for the Spleen to extract and distribute nutrients effectively. Eating in moderation (85% full) is recommended.

Alcohol consumption can deplete Qi and Blood, especially when consumed excessively. Moderation is key, and it's essential to stay hydrated if you choose to drink alcohol.

Coffee and caffeinated beverages have a drying effect on the body and may contribute to Qi and Blood Deficiency when consumed in excess.

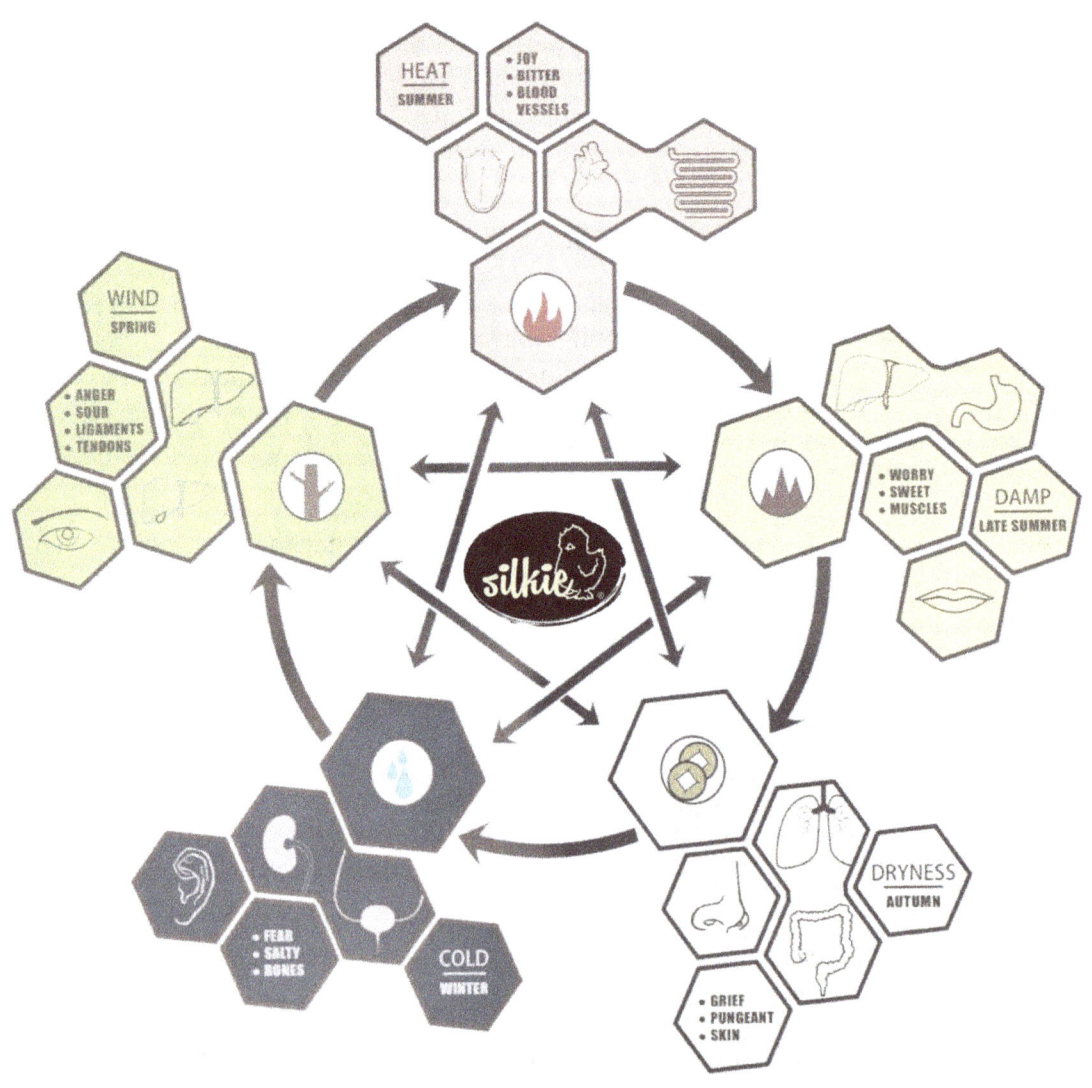

8. Floating Stool - Sign of Spleen Qi Deficiency without Dampness

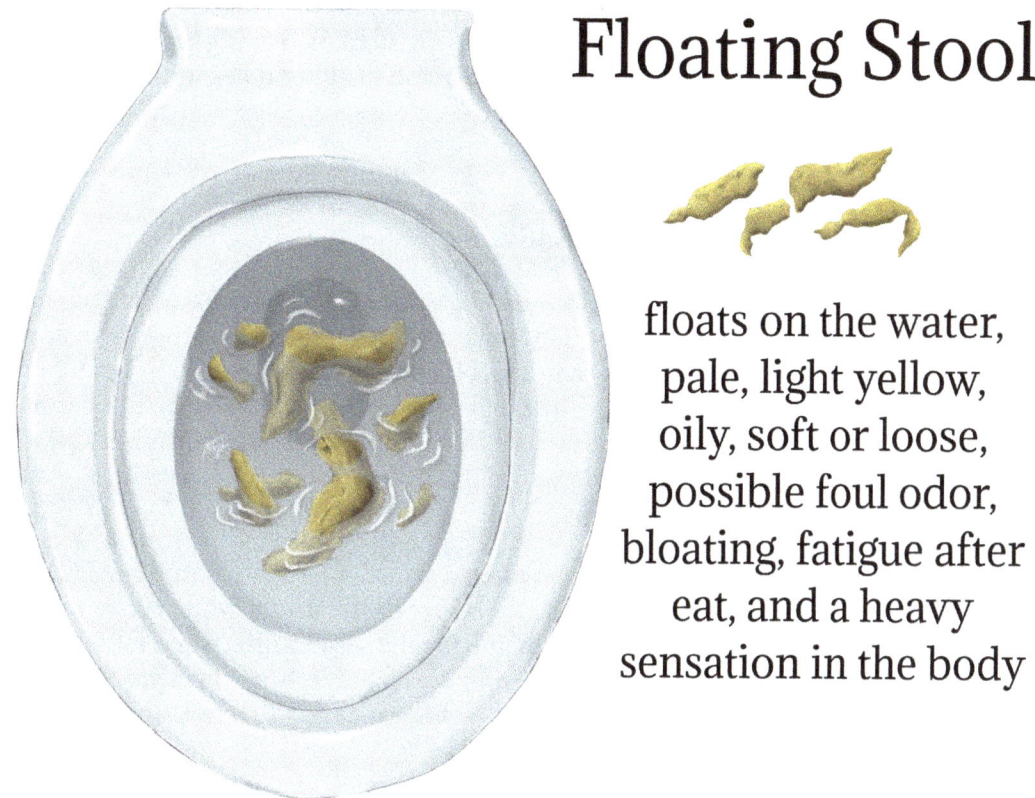

Floating Stool

floats on the water, pale, light yellow, oily, soft or loose, possible foul odor, bloating, fatigue after eat, and a heavy sensation in the body

Figure 6.8 Floating stool, Spleen Qi Deficiency, Liver and Spleen Disharmony without Dampness, Poor Fat Digestion.

What it Means: Floating stool usually indicates incomplete digestion, most often related to poor fat metabolism. In TCM, this reflects weakness in the Spleen's ability to transform and transport food, often complicated by dysfunction in the Liver and Gallbladder, where bile secretion is impaired and fats remain undigested. Because fats are lighter than water, they cause stool to float rather than sink, often leaving a greasy film on the toilet water or making the stool difficult to flush. In Western medicine, this corresponds to fat malabsorption, often linked to reduced bile production, impaired bile flow, or insufficient pancreatic enzyme activity.

Underlying Causes

If you've ever felt sluggish, bloated, or experienced ongoing digestive issues, the root cause may be Spleen Qi Deficiency with impaired fat transformation. The Spleen in TCM is responsible for extracting nutrients from food and converting them into Qi and Blood. When its function is weak, digestion slows and nutrients are only partially absorbed, leaving undigested residue in the stool. Greasy, fried, or overly sweet foods are the most common culprits, as they burden the Spleen and weaken its transformative fire. Cold or raw foods can further extinguish digestive warmth, leading to poor appetite, fatigue, and stools that are oily or buoyant.

The Liver and Gallbladder also play a critical role. The Liver ensures the smooth flow of Qi, while the Gallbladder stores and releases bile to help break down fats. When Liver Qi stagnates — often from stress, irregular eating, or emotional strain — bile secretion is impaired. Without sufficient bile, fats pass through undigested, leading to floating stools, oily films in the water, or stools that are difficult to flush. This shows how the Spleen's weakness and the Liver/Gallbladder's dysfunction combine to disrupt fat metabolism.

Other contributors include late-night meals, overeating, eating under stress, and sedentary living, all of which slow Qi circulation and weaken digestion. Chronic illness or long-term medication use may further sap the body's vitality, compounding poor fat absorption.

Floating stool can also arise from late-night meals, overeating, or eating under stress, which further strain the Spleen and upset Liver Qi flow. A sedentary lifestyle weakens Qi circulation, slowing digestion. Chronic illness or long-term use of certain medications may sap the body's vitality and disrupt fat absorption. Even environmental influences — such as prolonged exposure to damp climates — can weaken digestion and make the body more prone to malabsorption.

How Spleen Qi Deficiency Can Affect Our Body

When Spleen Qi becomes deficient, the entire body suffers. Digestion slows, nutrients aren't extracted efficiently, and the body lacks the energy to function optimally. This can manifest as fatigue, bloating, poor appetite, abdominal discomfort, and even loose or floating stools. Over time, because the Spleen also supports Blood production, deficiency may lead to pale complexion, dizziness, brittle nails, or hair loss. The partnership between the Spleen and Liver/Gallbladder is key here: a weak Spleen fails to transform food, while stagnant Liver Qi blocks bile flow, and together they impair fat metabolism. The result is stools that float and carry oily residue — clear signs that digestion is compromised.

In both TCM and Western terms, floating stool is most often a signal of fat malabsorption. TCM identifies this as a combination of Spleen Qi Deficiency and Liver/Gallbladder dysfunction, while Western medicine points to impaired bile or enzyme activity. Both perspectives highlight the same truth: when fat is not broken down properly, it passes into the stool, leaving behind oily, floating waste. Addressing this requires strengthening the Spleen, regulating Liver Qi, and supporting proper bile flow — a holistic approach to restoring digestive harmony.

Different Individuals May Experience Different Symptoms With Floating Stool

Digestive Discomfort. Bloating, fullness after meals, abdominal distention.

Greasy or Difficult-to-Flush Stool. Clear sign of fat malabsorption.

Fatigue. The Spleen's function of extracting nutrients from food and turning them into Qi and Blood are compromised. As a result, individuals may experience fatigue, weakness, and a lack of energy.

Weight Gain. Dampness tends to accumulate in the body, often leading to weight gain or difficulty losing weight. This is because the Spleen's ability to metabolize and transport fluids and nutrients is impaired.

Edema. Excess Dampness can manifest as edema or swelling in the limbs, particularly in the lower legs and ankles.

Mucus and Phlegm. Spleen Qi deficiency can lead to the production of excess mucus and phlegm. This can result in symptoms like a chronic cough, congestion, and a sensation of a lump in the throat. It may also cause the formation of painless, doughy lumps under the skin, commonly found around the neck, arms, or shoulders.

Brain Fog and Mental Fatigue. Qi deficiency can affect mental clarity and lead to cognitive issues, such as difficulty concentrating, forgetfulness, and mental fatigue.

Weakened Immunity. The Spleen plays a role in the body's immune system. When its Qi is deficient, individuals may be more susceptible to frequent illnesses.

Muscle Weakness. Weakness in the muscles and limbs can occur due to a lack of Qi nourishing the muscles.

Heavy Limbs. Individuals may experience a sensation of heaviness in the limbs, making physical activities more challenging.

Cold Limbs. Spleen Qi deficiency can lead to poor circulation and a feeling of coldness, especially in the extremities.

Prolonged Recovery. Injuries and illnesses may take longer to heal and recover from due to reduced Qi and nutrient availability.

Emotional Imbalance. Spleen Qi deficiency can lead to overthinking, worry, and mental fatigue. When Liver Qi stagnation is also present, irritability, mood swings, and emotional instability may occur.

Self-Care and Support

1. **Eat warm, cooked foods.** Focus on well-cooked, warm, and easily digestible meals. Avoid or minimize raw, cold, and greasy foods.

2. **Emphasize whole grains.** Incorporate grains like rice, oats, and quinoa into your diet as they are easier on the Spleen.

3. **Cook with digestive herbs.** Use herbs and spices like ginger, cinnamon, and fennel to aid digestion.

4. **Limit dairy and sweets.** Reduce the intake of dairy products and sugary foods, as they can contribute to dampness.

5. **Eat smaller meals.** Instead of large meals, opt for 4–6 smaller meals spaced throughout the day to ease the digestive burden on the Spleen. This approach helps maintain steady energy, supports smoother digestion, and prevents overtaxing the Spleen Qi.

6. **Get herbal remedies.** Consult a qualified TCM practitioner for herbal formulas specifically tailored to your condition. Common herbs for this pattern may include codonopsis, atractylodes, magnolia bark and poria.

Lifestyle Adjustments

1. **Manage stress.** Stress can weaken the Spleen. Incorporate stress-reduction techniques like meditation, deep breathing, and mindfulness.

2. **Get regular exercise.** Gentle, moderate exercise, such as walking or Tai Chi, can promote better circulation and support digestion.

3. **Maintain regular eating habits.** Eating meals at consistent times each day can help the Spleen's function.

4. **Avoid overeating.** Overloading the digestive system can worsen dampness. Practice portion control.

5. **Keep the abdominal area warm.** The Spleen is sensitive to cold, so dress warmly and use heating pads if necessary.

6. **Stay hydrated.** Drink warm beverages like ginger tea. Avoid excessive cold or iced drinks.

7. **Avoid damp environments.** Minimize exposure to damp and humid conditions, which can exacerbate dampness in the body.

8. **Rest and sleep.** Ensure you get sufficient rest and sleep, as fatigue can weaken the Spleen further.

9. **Apply acupressure.** Self-acupressure techniques can be learned for symptom relief. The Spleen-6 (SP6) or Stomach 36 (ST36) points are often used for digestive issues.

Foods To Relieve Spleen Qi Deficiency With Or Without Dampness

Cooked grains. Whole grains like rice, oats, and quinoa are easy on the Spleen and provide a good source of energy.

Root vegetables. Sweet potatoes, carrots, and squash are grounding and help tonify the Spleen.

Lean proteins. Lean meats like chicken, pork tenderloin, and fish are easier to digest than fatty cuts and help support the Spleen. Plant-based proteins like tofu and tempeh are generally cooling in nature and can weaken the Spleen if eaten regularly, especially when digestion is already compromised. For now, it's best to avoid them until the Spleen is stronger.

Vegetables. Cooked, well-cooked vegetables are easier on the digestive system than raw ones. Consider options like zucchini, green beans, and carrots.

Fruits. Fruits should be eaten in moderation. Cooked or stewed fruits, such as apples or pears, are gentler on the Spleen. Avoid excessive consumption of cold or tropical fruits.

Warming spices. Incorporate spices like ginger, cinnamon, and fennel into your cooking. These can help stimulate digestion.

Congee. This rice porridge is a traditional Chinese remedy for digestive issues. You can customize it with various ingredients, including lean meats, vegetables, and seasonings.

Bone broth. Homemade bone broth is nourishing and supportive of the digestive system. It provides essential nutrients and is gentle on the Spleen.

Soups and stews. These are easy to digest and can be prepared with Spleen-friendly ingredients like root vegetables, lean protein, and warming spices.

Herbs. Herbs to strengthen the Spleen, resolve Dampness, and improve transformation include Chinese Yam (Shan Yao), Lotus Seed (Lian Zi), Job's Tears (Yi Yi Ren), and Atractylodes Rhizome (Bai Zhu). It is best to work with a qualified TCM practitioner when using herbal formulas. For daily support, herbal teas made with roasted barley, coix seed, and tangerine peel are helpful.

Nuts and seeds. Small amounts of almonds, walnuts, and pumpkin seeds can be included in your diet as snacks.

Fermented foods (in moderation). Small amounts of fermented foods like sauerkraut may help promote a healthy gut, but not dairy products like cold yogurt or kefir.

Proper food combining. Avoid combining foods that may create digestive issues. For example, try not to consume fruit immediately after a heavy meal. Many Chinese restaurants serve orange slices after a meal because they're refreshing, lightly sweet, and help cleanse the palate after oily dishes. In TCM, the sweet–slightly sour nature of oranges can promote Qi flow and aid digestion, especially in moving greasy food through the system. However, from a digestive standpoint, eating raw fruit right after a heavy meal can burden the Spleen and slow digestion, so it's best enjoyed in moderation or after some time has passed rather than immediately.

Foods That Can Worsen Spleen Qi Deficiency With Or Without Dampness

Cold foods, drinks and damp-producing foods. Stay away from foods that can exacerbate Dampness and weaken the Spleen. This includes cold drinks, ice cream, foods straight from the refrigerator, dairy, and greasy or fried foods.

Raw foods. Excessive consumption of raw fruits and vegetables, especially in a cold climate, may stress the Spleen. It's better to cook or lightly steam them.

Dairy products. Dairy can be hard to digest and easily produces mucus, thereby potentially worsening Spleen Qi Deficiency.

Excessive sugary foods. Overconsumption of sugary foods and drinks lead to dampness and mucus, which exacerbates the Spleen's condition.

Fried or greasy foods. These can be difficult for the Spleen to process and when consumed regularly or in large quantities lead to dampness and mucus.

Excessive caffeine. Coffee and caffeinated beverages can have a dehydrating effect and weaken the Spleen over time.

Alcohol. Excessive alcohol consumption can create dampness and heat in the body, further taxing the Spleen.

Spicy foods. While some warming spices can help the Spleen, excessively spicy or hot foods generate dampness and heat.

Heavy meals. Large, heavy meals can overwhelm the Spleen. Smaller, more frequent meals are often better.

Processed and refined foods. Processed foods with artificial additives and preservatives are challenging for the digestive system.

Excessive sweeteners. Artificial sweeteners or excessive sugar consumption contribute to dampness.

Too much salt. Excessive salt intake can lead to fluid retention and may worsen dampness.

Iced drinks. Extremely cold or iced drinks can weaken the digestive process.

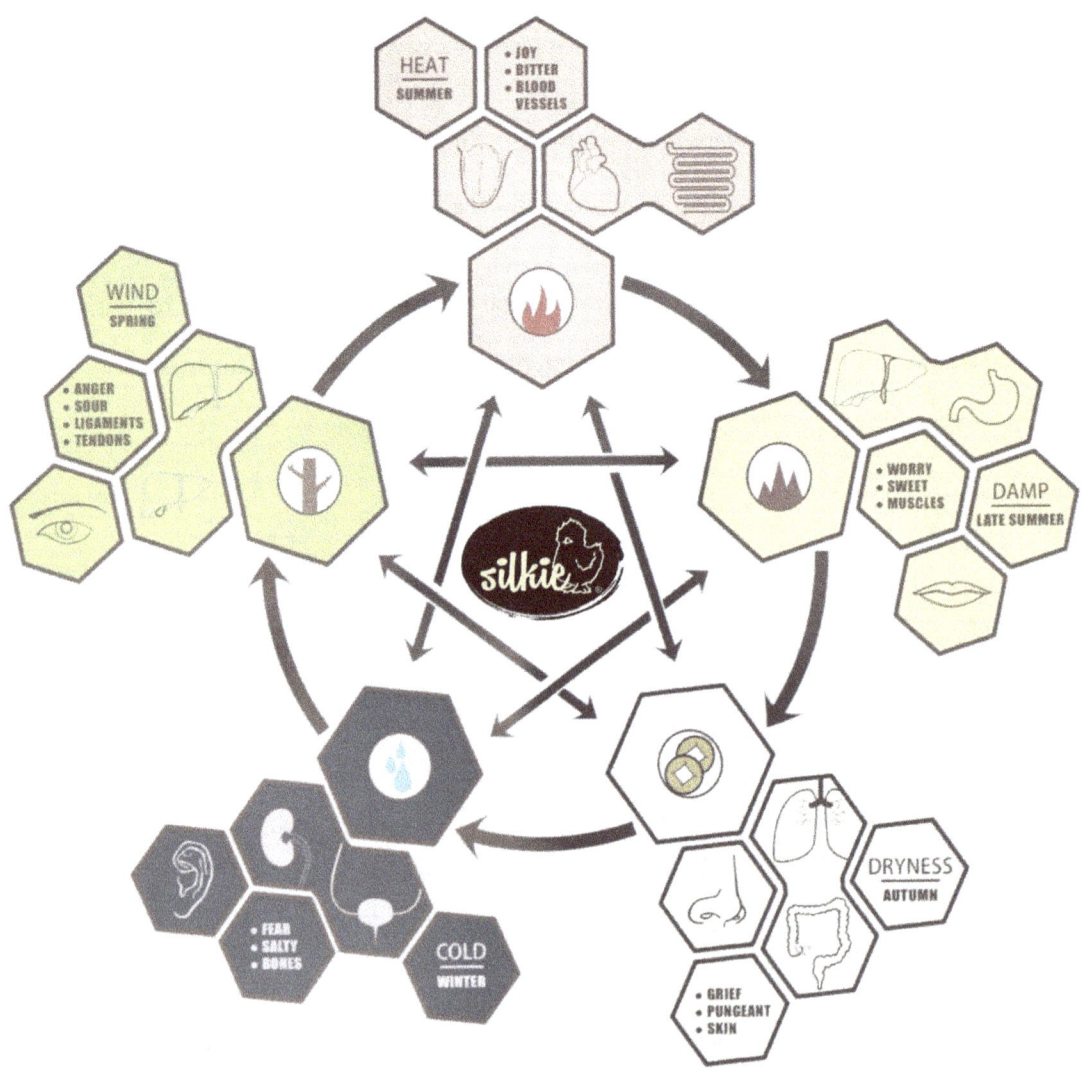

9. Sinking & Sticky Stool – Sign of Dampness blocking the Spleen

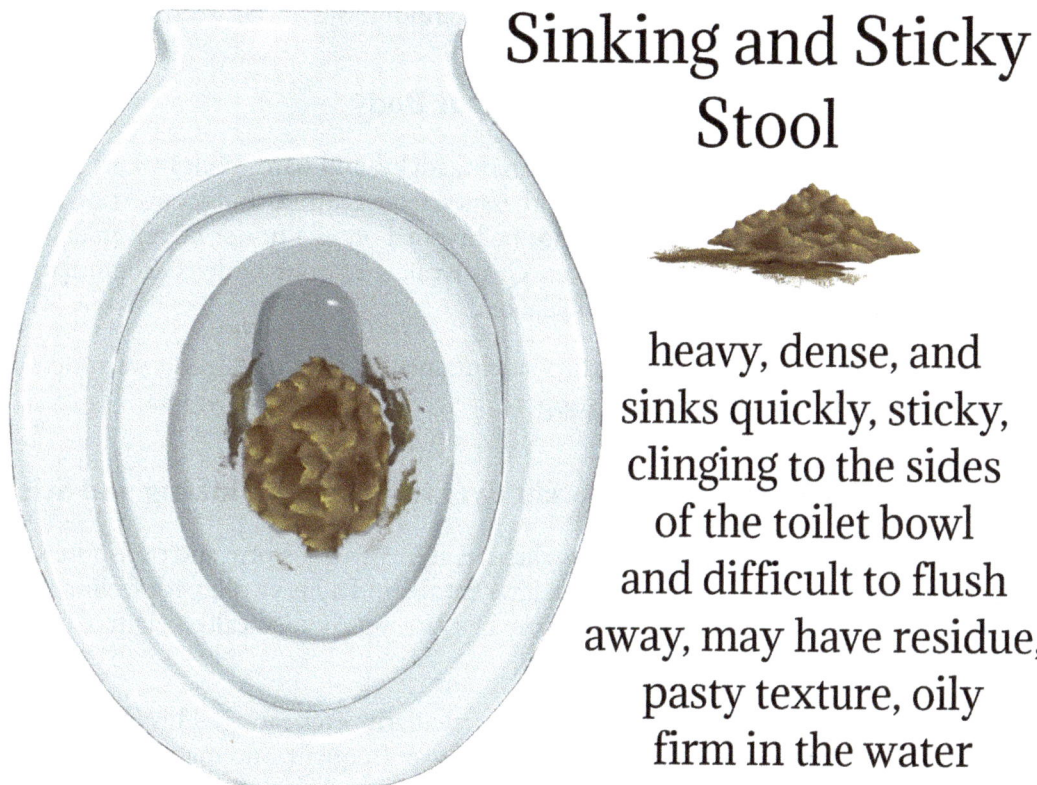

Sinking and Sticky Stool

heavy, dense, and sinks quickly, sticky, clinging to the sides of the toilet bowl and difficult to flush away, may have residue, pasty texture, oily firm in the water

Figure 6.9 Sinking and sticky stool, Dampness blocking the Spleen.

What It Means: When stool sinks heavily to the bottom of the toilet and clings to the sides, leaving residue that is difficult to flush, it usually indicates Dampness obstructing the Spleen's function. In TCM, Dampness is not just water but a pathological byproduct that forms when the Spleen cannot properly transform and transport fluids. Instead of sending nutrients upward and waste downward, the Spleen's weakened Qi leaves fluids stagnating, thickening, and mixing with waste. This creates stools that are dense, sticky, and heavy.

Unlike floating stools, which result from undigested fats and poor bile function, sinking sticky stools are weighed down by Dampness. It is as though the body's metabolism has slowed, unable to burn off excess moisture, leaving behind tacky residue that makes stools pasty and difficult to pass cleanly.

Underlying Causes

The main drivers of this condition often come from dietary and lifestyle habits. Greasy, oily foods, fried dishes, fatty meats, and overly sweet desserts are classic Dampness-producing culprits. Excessive intake of raw salads, iced drinks, or smoothies further extinguishes the digestive warmth the Spleen needs to function properly. Overeating, eating irregularly, or late-night meals weaken the digestive system further, while sedentary living reduces Qi circulation and makes it harder to metabolize fluids. Emotional strain, especially worry and overthinking, which directly affect the Spleen, can also contribute to this imbalance.

Environmental Dampness, such as humid weather, damp living spaces, or prolonged exposure to moisture, may seep inward and aggravate the body's internal Dampness, creating a cycle where the Spleen is too weak to resolve it and the Dampness, in turn, weighs the Spleen down even more. Sticky stools rarely appear alone and are often accompanied by other symptoms. Many people with this condition feel a sensation of heaviness in their body or limbs, fatigue and sluggishness that worsens after meals, bloating, poor appetite, and even brain fog or difficulty concentrating. They may also produce excess mucus or phlegm, notice swelling in their legs or ankles, or feel mentally cloudy and physically weighed down. A greasy tongue coating, either white or yellow depending on whether Cold or Heat combines with Dampness, is another classic sign. Together, these clues paint a picture of a metabolism bogged down by unresolved fluids that the Spleen cannot move or transform efficiently.

How Dampness Blocking The Spleen Can Affect Our Body

In TCM, Dampness is often compared to a swamp: stagnant, sticky, and hard to clear. Left unchecked, it can transform into Phlegm and cause more complicated health issues, from chronic sinus congestion to cysts, lipomas and masses. That is why sinking, sticky stool should not be brushed off as a minor inconvenience. It is an early warning that your digestion is struggling, your Spleen Qi is weak, and your body is accumulating unwanted Dampness that can spread and cause more serious imbalances.

That's why sticky, sinking stools are not just a bathroom nuisance — they're an early warning sign that your metabolism is bogged down and your Spleen needs support.

Different Individuals May Experience Different Symptoms With Sinking and Sticky Stool

Digestive Issues. Dampness obstructing the Spleen weakens its ability to transform and transport food and fluids. This often shows up as bloating, abdominal distension after meals, and a heavy, sluggish feeling in the stomach. Stools are dense, sticky, and difficult to flush. Appetite may be poor, yet paradoxically weight may increase due to inefficient metabolism.

Fatigue. Individuals commonly feel sluggish and drained, particularly after eating. This is because the Spleen is not transforming food into sufficient Qi and Blood. Energy dips are frequent, and many report a heavy, lethargic feeling throughout the day.

Heaviness in the Body. Dampness creates a sense of weight, especially in the limbs. This heaviness is not due to muscle weakness but from obstructed Qi circulation and fluid retention.

Mucus and Phlegm. Excess Dampness often transforms into Phlegm. This may appear as sinus congestion, frequent throat clearing, thick saliva, or postnasal drip. Some individuals also notice phlegm-related coughs or chest congestion. It may also cause the formation of painless, doughy lumps found under the skin.

Brain Fog and Poor Concentration. Dampness clouds the mind, leading to mental heaviness, forgetfulness, or difficulty focusing. This mental swampiness is a common companion to digestive sluggishness.

Swelling and Edema. Damp accumulation often manifests as swelling, especially in the lower extremities like the legs and ankles. This reflects the Spleen's inability to regulate fluids properly.

Tongue and Pulse Signs. In TCM diagnosis, a thick, greasy tongue coating is common — white if Cold-Damp predominates, yellow if Heat-Damp predominates. The pulse is often slippery, reflecting the body's burden of unresolved Dampness.

Self-Care and Support

Gentle Exercise. Engage in tai chi, qi gong, brisk walking, or light movement to circulate Qi and fluids.

Manage Emotions. Overthinking and worry directly tax the Spleen. Breathing exercises, meditation, or journaling can help ease mental strain.

Professional Treatment. Acupuncture and customized herbal formulas prescribed by a TCM practitioner can tonify the Spleen and resolve Dampness.

Routine. Establish regular mealtimes and avoid late-night eating to reduce digestive strain.

Foods To Relieve Spleen Block By Dampness

Warm, cooked grains. Millet, oats, and rice porridge (congee) gently strengthen the Spleen and aid digestion. Because they are soft, warm, and easy to break down, they supply steady energy while preventing the build-up of excess fluids that contribute to Dampness.

Light soups and stews. Barley soup, mung bean soup (for Heat-Damp), or chicken/bone broth with root vegetables support hydration while promoting transformation. These meals are easy to digest, restore warmth, and help the body clear heaviness without overburdening the Spleen.

Spleen-strengthening foods. Chinese yam, lotus seeds, red dates, pumpkin, carrots, and sweet potatoes help tonify Qi and nourish digestion. They provide natural sweetness that supports the Spleen, while their warm, grounding nature offsets Dampness and sluggish metabolism.

Aromatic herbs and spices. Ginger, cardamom, fennel, cinnamon, and clove invigorate digestion by warming the center and dispersing stagnant fluids. Their fragrance moves Qi, helping prevent bloating, heaviness, and the sticky residue that Dampness leaves in the body.

Legumes (in moderation). Adzuki beans, lentils, and other small beans strengthen digestion and help drain Dampness. Well-cooked legumes provide fiber and nutrients while avoiding heaviness, supporting both energy production and fluid balance.

Mild teas. Ginger tea warms digestion and revives Qi, poria tea drains Dampness, and light barley tea relieves bloating and heaviness. These teas are gentle daily options that complement meals and restore clarity to digestion.

Herbs. Herbs to dry Dampness, strengthen the Spleen, and improve digestive transformation include Poria (Fu Ling), Atractylodes Rhizome (Bai Zhu), Magnolia Bark (Hou Po), and Agastache (Huo Xiang). It is best to work with a qualified TCM practitioner when using herbal formulas.

Foods That Can Worsen Spleen Block By Dampness

Greasy and oily foods. Fried dishes, fatty meats, and heavy oils create Damp residues that the Spleen struggles to transform. Over time, they lead to sticky stools, bloating, and heaviness in the limbs.

Excess sugar and sweets. Refined sugar, pastries, and desserts weaken Spleen Qi, producing sticky Dampness. Too much sweetness also encourages cravings, further draining the digestive system.

Cold and raw foods. Raw salads, sushi, iced drinks, and smoothies weaken the digestive fire and slow nutrient transformation. They easily overwhelm a weak Spleen, leading to bloating and loose stools.

Damp-forming foods. Dairy (milk, cheese, yogurt), bananas, melons, and cucumbers generate excess moisture in the gut. These foods can create mucus, heaviness, and cloudy thinking when digestion is weak.

Alcohol and excessive coffee. Alcohol adds Damp-Heat that burdens the Liver and Spleen, while overuse of coffee scatters Qi and irritates digestion. Both worsen bloating, heaviness, and Damp stagnation.

Highly processed foods. Fast food, packaged snacks, and processed meats lack vitality and are hard to digest. They stagnate Qi, produce internal Dampness, and leave the body sluggish and heavy.

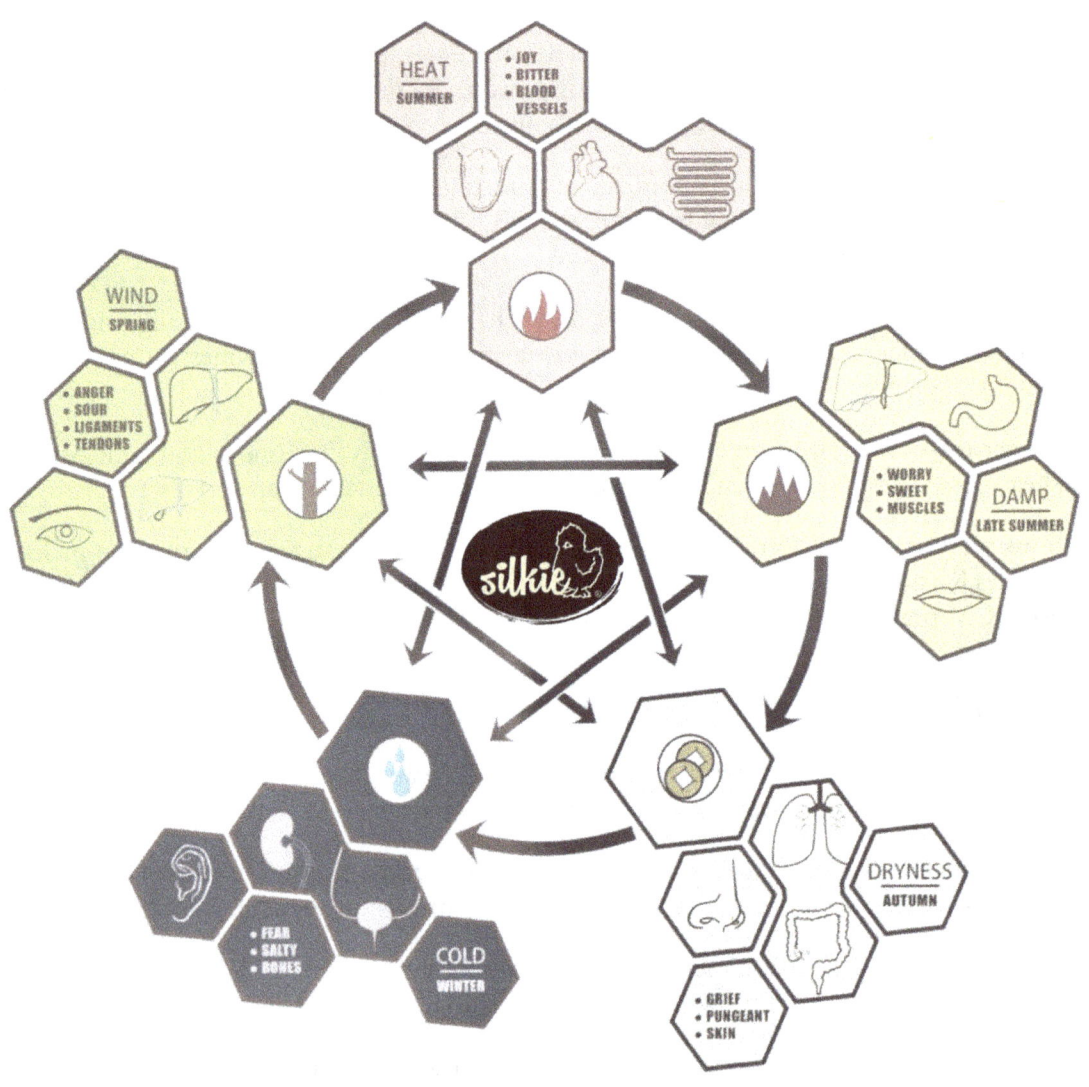

10. Dry, Hard, Dark Pebbles That Are Hard To Pass - Indicative of Blood Dryness due to prolonged Deficiency in Qi and Blood

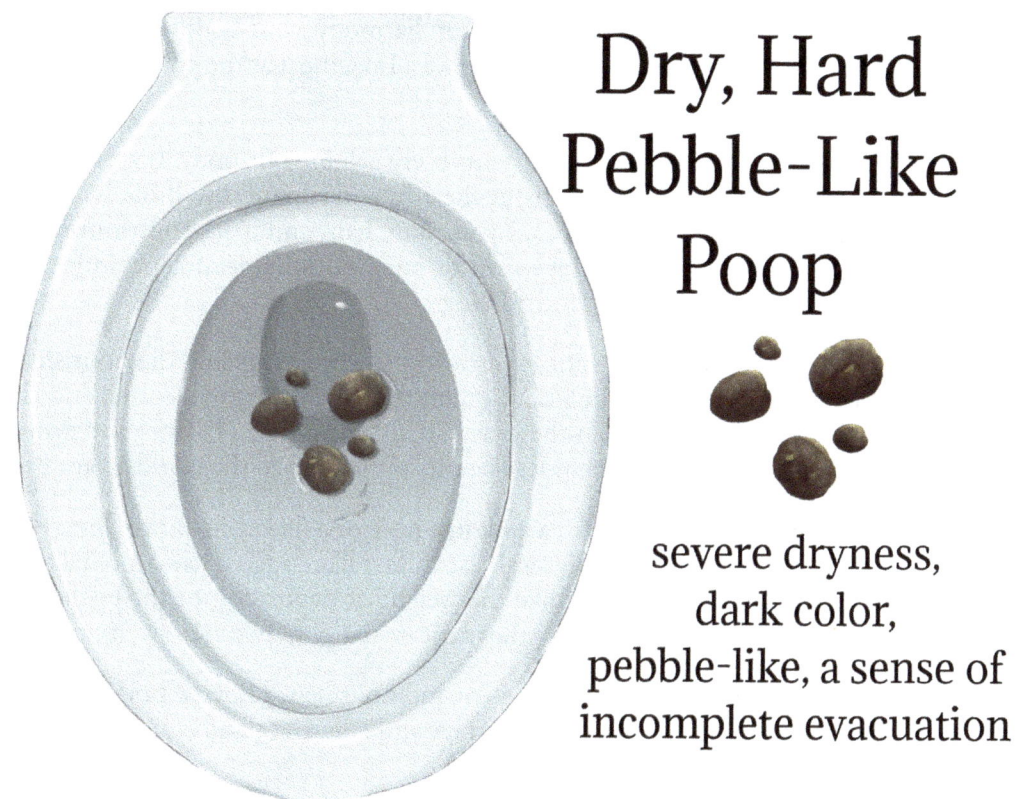

Figure 6.10 Dry, hard, pebble-like poop, prolonged Blood and Qi Deficiency, Blood Dryness, Severe Dryness and Stagnation in the Large Intestine.

What It Means: If your poop is very dry, hard, and pebble-like, similar to goat droppings, and you struggle to pass it or feel the urge to go but can't, then this is indicative of long term Qi and Blood Deficiency leading to the condition of Blood Dryness. Common symptoms of Blood Dryness are dry and flaky skin, dry and brittle hair, chapped and dry lips, dry and hard stools, or drinking fluids but still feeling dry.

Underlying Causes

Qi and Blood are essential elements in traditional Chinese medicine that provide energy and nourishment to the body. A deficiency in these vital substances can lead to various health issues, including digestive problems. Chronic Qi and Blood deficiency can lead to Blood Dryness. This is a condition where the Blood lacks sufficient moisture to nourish the body and keep it from drying out. Blood Dryness can be caused by various factors such as dietary imbalances, severe or prolonged illness, or trauma resulting in heavy blood loss.

Blood Dryness is quite common in postpartum recovery. After childbirth, women may experience hard, dry, pebbly stools if they haven't fully regained their Qi and Blood. Experiencing severe or frequent morning sickness during pregnancy often leads to pebble-like stools after giving birth. This is because persistent vomiting and reduced food and fluid intake during pregnancy can deplete the body's fluids and disrupt the digestive system's normal function, potentially contributing to drier, harder stools postpartum. Other factors such as having a history of prolonged stress, overworking or over exercising, a history of being vegan or vegetarian or long periods of not sleeping well through the night can cause dry, hard, pebbly stools.

The Importance of Blood and Qi in the Body

Step into the fascinating world of Traditional Chinese Medicine, where the secrets to vibrant health lie in understanding two fundamental treasures: Qi and Blood. Think of Qi as the very spark of life within you, the vital energy that animates every single function, from the tireless work of digestion to the lightning-fast connections of your thoughts. It's the invisible force that ensures your organs hum in harmony, your bodily fluids flow smoothly, and you have the get-up-and-go for everything the day throws your way. Imagine it as the power source that keeps your internal systems running.

Now, picture Blood as the rich, nourishing elixir that sustains every cell in your body. It's the vital fluid carrying essential nutrients and life-giving oxygen, keeping your tissues healthy and vibrant. But Blood's role extends beyond mere delivery; it's also the deep wellspring of moisture for your skin, hair, and nails, contributing to that healthy glow. Interestingly, in TCM, Blood is also deeply connected to our emotional landscape, influencing our inner sense of calm and well-being. Blood nourishes your entire being.

In essence, Qi and Blood are the dynamic duo of your inner world — the energy and the nourishment that keep everything, from the tiniest cellular activity to the grand orchestra of your organ systems and the strength of your muscles, functioning in perfect rhythm. When these two are in harmonious balance and flowing freely, you experience a profound sense of internal integration and a vibrant connection to the world around you.

However, when this delicate balance is disrupted, like a kink in a hose or a flickering power line, symptoms begin to surface. These can manifest in a myriad of ways: physical discomfort like nagging pain, mental fog or even more severe cognitive challenges, or emotional turbulence like the weight of depression or the restlessness of anxiety. This is why TCM takes a holistic approach, recognizing the intricate dance between body, mind, and emotions.

Ultimately, the key to robust health lies in ensuring a sufficient and unimpeded flow of both Qi and Blood. When these two are in perfect harmony, your body operates with grace and efficiency, and you feel resilient and capable of navigating life's demands with ease.

Conversely, imbalances — whether it's an excess, a deficiency, or a stagnation of either Qi or Blood — are seen as the root of "dis-ease," affecting not just the physical body but also the mind and spirit. Like skilled detectives, TCM practitioners employ a range of diagnostic tools to uncover these imbalances. They might carefully observe the subtle cues in your face and eyes, feel the intricate rhythms of your pulse, examine the landscape of your tongue, gently palpate your abdomen and limbs, and listen attentively to your detailed account of your symptoms. Sometimes a single method provides the key, while other times a combination paints a more complete picture. The goal of TCM treatments, whether through the strategic placement of acupuncture needles, the carefully crafted formulas of herbal medicine, or the nourishing wisdom of food therapy, is always to gently guide Qi and Blood back into their natural balance, addressing the very root of any health concerns and restoring your innate vitality.

Different Individuals May Experience Different Symptoms With Pebble-like Poop

Abdominal Discomfort. This condition might also come with sensations of fullness in your chest and upper abdomen, frequent belching, a reduced appetite, and occasional abdominal discomfort, and bloating.

Fatigue. Individuals may experience persistent fatigue, weakness or dizziness, often described as a lack of energy. This fatigue may affect daily activities and overall vitality.

Pale Complexion. A pale or sallow complexion can be an external sign of Blood Deficiency. The skin may appear dull and lacking in luster.

Pale Lips and Nails. Lips and nails may appear pale, lacking their natural color.

Dry Skin and Hair. Dry and flaky skin, as well as brittle and dry hair, are common manifestations of Blood Deficiency and Dryness.

Brittle Nails. Nails may become brittle, prone to cracking, and have a pale appearance.

Dry Eyes and Blurred Vision. Dryness of the eyes and blurred vision may occur due to a lack of Blood to nourish and moisten the eyes.

Dry and Cracked Tongue. A pale, dry, cracked tongue is common with Blood Deficiency and Dryness.

Dizziness and Lightheadedness. Individuals may experience dizziness or lightheadedness, especially when standing up quickly.

Palpitations. Heart palpitations or an awareness of one's heartbeat may occur, often accompanied by a sensation of "emptiness" in the chest.

Shortness of Breath. Some individuals may have difficulty catching their breath or experience shortness of breath, even with minimal physical exertion.

Poor Memory and Concentration. Cognitive symptoms such as forgetfulness, poor memory, and difficulty concentrating are associated with Blood Deficiency.

Insomnia. Difficulty falling asleep or staying asleep may be a symptom of Blood Deficiency.

Numbness and Tingling. Numbness, tingling, or a "pins and needles" sensation in the extremities can occur.

Irregular Menstrual Cycles. In women, Blood Deficiency can lead to irregular menstrual cycles, light (scanty) menstrual flow, or amenorrhea (absence of menstruation).

Tinnitus. Ringing or buzzing in the ears (tinnitus) can sometimes be related to Blood Deficiency.

Cold Extremities. Blood Deficiency is often associated with a lack of warmth or vitality, therefore, some individuals may experience cold hands or feet.

Mood Swings or Emotional Imbalances. Anger, anxiety, depression, sadness, worry, and crying for no reason can be symptoms of Blood Deficiency.

Self-Care and Support

Rest and Recovery. Adequate rest and recovery are crucial for individuals in this situation. The body needs time to replenish Qi and Blood.

Nutrient-Rich Diet. Consuming a diet rich in nutrients, including foods like bone broth, can help nourish and support Qi and Blood production. These nutrient-dense foods provide essential vitamins and minerals that contribute to overall health.

Hydration. Staying well-hydrated is crucial to address dryness in the body, including digestive tract dryness. Sufficient hydration supports overall bodily functions. Try to drink as much water as you can between 7 am and 7 pm. Try to sip your water throughout the day.

Water Plus 1 Drop of Honey. Honey water is for those who drink a lot of water but pee it all out and still feel dry and thirsty. Do not use a lot of honey. Too much honey may increase your risk of diabetes.

Foods To Relieve Blood Dryness And Deficiency In Qi And Blood

Angelica Sinensis (Dang Gui). This herb is highly regarded in TCM for its Blood-nourishing properties. It is often used to address Blood Deficiency and regulate menstruation.

Goji berries (Gou Qi Zi). Goji berries are often referred to as a "superfood." They nourish the Liver and Kidneys, support vision, and boost overall vitality.

Chinese red dates (Hong Zao). Red dates are rich in nutrients and are used to tonify Qi and Blood, making them beneficial for those with Qi and Blood Deficiency. Moderate intake (about 3 dates per day) is recommended.

Longan (Long Yan Rou). Longan fruit is known for its ability to strengthen the Spleen, nourish the Blood, and calm the mind. Longan should be paired with dragon fruit or mangosteen, because longan can be too Yang (warming) when eaten alone.

Chinese black dates (Hei Zao). Black dates are used to nourish the Blood, support digestion, and promote Qi circulation. Moderate intake (about 3 dates per day) is recommended.

Black mulberry (Sang Shen Zi). These berries are similar to goji berries and nourish the Liver and Kidneys, improve vision, and enhance overall vitality. Moderate intake (about 3 - 5 pieces per day) is recommended.

Dragon fruit. Moderate intake of dragon fruit is considered cooling in TCM and can help balance excess internal heat. It is often used to soothe dryness and inflammation.

Red and dark colored fruits and vegetables. Berries, like blueberries, blackberries, strawberries, are rich in antioxidants and can help support overall blood health. Beets are high in iron, which is essential for blood production, and they can help combat Blood Deficiency.

Leafy greens. Spinach, kale, and other leafy greens are excellent sources of folate, which is essential for the production of red blood cells and can help address Blood Deficiency. These leafy greens should be cooked for better digestion and absorption.

Lean proteins. Lean meats, poultry, fish, and tofu provide essential amino acids required for building and maintaining both Qi and Blood.

Legumes. Beans, lentils, and chickpeas are rich in iron, protein, and fiber. They support Qi and Blood production and are useful for vegetarians and vegans.

Whole grains. Whole grains like white rice, brown rice, quinoa, and oats provide sustained energy and support Qi and Blood nourishment.

Bone broth. Bone broth contains essential nutrients like collagen, which supports Blood and Qi. It is also hydrating and can help with overall vitality.

TCM soups and stews. Traditional Chinese medicine often incorporates herbal soups and stews with ingredients like Chinese goji berries and ginseng, which nourish Qi and Blood.

Herbs. Herbs to nourish Blood, moisten the intestines, and improve elimination include Angelica Root (Dang Gui), Hemp Seed (Huo Ma Ren), and Rehmannia Root (Sheng Di Huang). It is best to work with a qualified TCM practitioner when using herbal formulas. For daily support, herbal teas made from Qi and Blood tonifying herbs like astragalus, red dates, and hibiscus are beneficial at the right dosages and combinations.

Adaptogenic herbs. Adaptogens like ashwagandha and astragalus can help the body adapt to stress and support overall vitality, including Qi and Blood.

Fruits high in vitamin C. Citrus fruits, kiwi, and guava provide vitamin C, which enhances iron absorption from plant-based sources.

Sesame seeds. Sesame seeds, particularly black sesame seeds, are considered nourishing for both Qi and Blood in TCM.

Liver-friendly foods. Foods that support the Liver such as bitter greens should be cooked before consuming. For example, small amounts of dandelion can indirectly benefit blood as the Liver plays a crucial role in Blood regulation.

Foods That Can Worsen Blood Dryness And Deficiency In Qi And Blood

Spicy foods, especially those with hot peppers and strong spices, can exacerbate internal heat and may contribute to dryness in the body.

Coffee and caffeinated beverages can have a drying effect on the body and may contribute to Qi and Blood Deficiency when consumed in excess.

Alcohol dehydrates and can lead to dryness in the body. Excessive alcohol consumption can affect the Liver and Blood, contributing to deficiencies.

High-sodium diets, often associated with processed and salty foods, can lead to excessive thirst and potentially disrupt fluid balance, exacerbating dryness.

Highly processed foods, especially those high in sugar, can have an inflammatory effect on the body and do not provide the nourishment needed to support Qi and Blood.

Excessive sweets lead to fluctuations in blood sugar levels and may not provide the sustained energy needed to support Qi and Blood.

Excessive raw and cold foods, especially in cold weather or for individuals who tend to feel cold easily, may interfere with digestion and lead to Dampness and Coldness.

Iced or cold beverages weaken the digestive system and potentially hinder Qi and Blood production and circulation.

Dairy consumption may contribute to phlegm and Dampness which block the flow of Qi and Blood.

Fried and greasy foods are heavy and contribute to sluggish digestion, potentially affecting nutrient absorption.

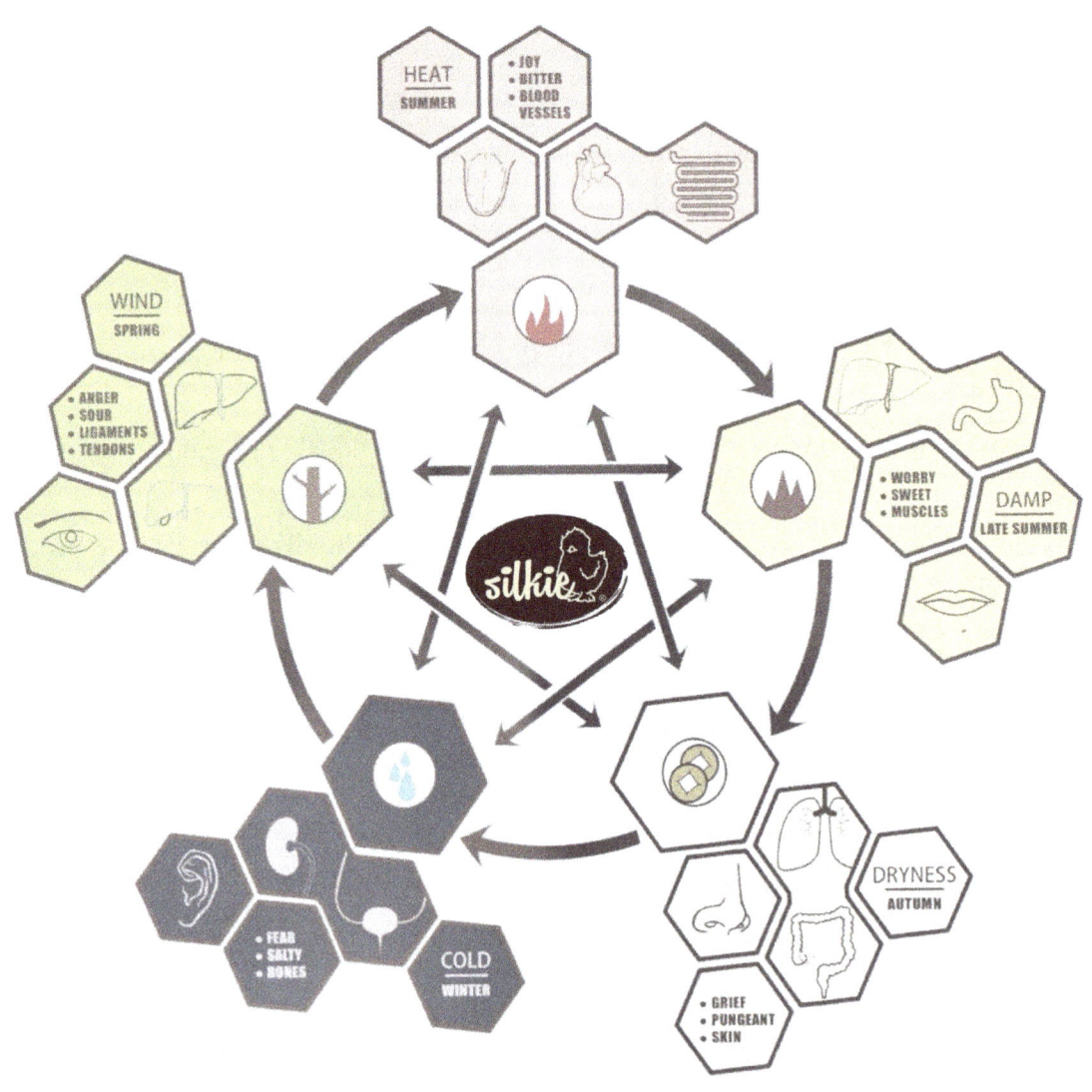

11. Dark To Light Watery Stool Multiple Times Within A Day With Rotten Odor- Sign of food retention or food poisoning

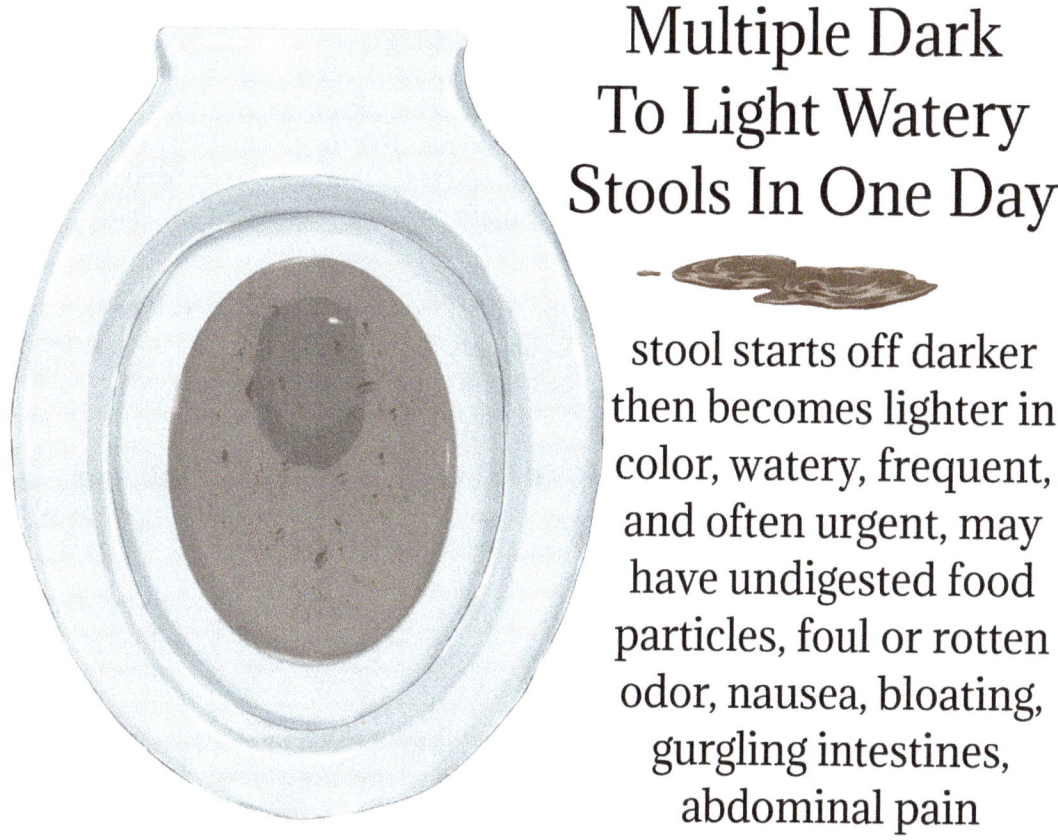

Multiple Dark To Light Watery Stools In One Day

stool starts off darker then becomes lighter in color, watery, frequent, and often urgent, may have undigested food particles, foul or rotten odor, nausea, bloating, gurgling intestines, abdominal pain

Figure 6.11 Dark to light multiple watery stools, Food Stagnation, Cold-Damp in the Intestines, or Toxic Heat attacking the Stomach and Spleen.

What it Means: When you experience dark to light brown, watery, and foul-smelling stools multiple times a day, particularly with no solid pieces, it's often a sign of Food Retention with Damp Heat, Cold-Damp in the Intestines, or Toxic Heat attacking the Stomach and Spleen. In Traditional Chinese Medicine, this indicates poor digestion, where food isn't being properly broken down and absorbed, often lingering too long in the digestive system. This can happen when spoiled or contaminated food (known as "Toxic Heat" in TCM) or excessive amounts of cold/raw foods lead to Stagnation and Damp Accumulation in the Stomach and Intestines.

When the body is trying to expel toxins or pathogenic factors quickly, it may result in multiple watery bowel movements. These may begin dark in color, reflecting accumulated waste and internal Heat or Damp-Heat, but gradually become lighter as the digestive system weakens and loses the strength to fully process and eliminate. The lighter color in this case is not necessarily a sign that toxins are gone, but rather that the Spleen and Stomach can no longer effectively transform waste or fluids, leading to dilution and poor elimination. The undigested food can generate internal Dampness and Heat, leading to the characteristic watery, strong-smelling stools. This dampness in the digestive tract can also cause uncomfortable symptoms like bloating, discomfort, and irregular bowel movements. This Food Retention often stems from consuming heavy, greasy, or otherwise hard-to-digest foods including toxic or spoiled foods causing an imbalance in your digestive process.

Underlying Causes

In Traditional Chinese Medicine, food retention isn't just about what you eat; it delves into *how* you eat and even your overall lifestyle. It happens when your digestive system struggles to efficiently break down and move food. This leads to a build-up that causes discomfort and a host of other issues.

When considering what we consume, several habits can pave the way for food retention. Overloading your system with heavy, rich, greasy, or fatty foods is a prime culprit, much like trying to push too much through a pipe. These foods create dampness and phlegm in the body, further gumming up the digestive machinery. This is why overeating at a buffet or on Thanksgiving day can also lead to food retention. It might seem obvious, but consuming contaminated or spoiled food can directly lead to digestive upset and retention; TCM emphasizes fresh, clean, and properly prepared food for good reason.

Ever wolf down a meal without properly chewing or mindful attention? This hinders digestion from the start, forcing your stomach to overwork and increasing the likelihood of food getting stuck. Likewise, raw foods can also hinder digestion. An abundance of cold or raw foods can weaken the digestive fire (Yang energy). This makes your Spleen, Stomach, and Intestines less effective at processing food.

Inconsistent eating habits, such as skipping meals or eating at irregular times, also disrupt your body's natural digestive rhythm. Your system thrives on regularity. Additionally, a diet lacking variety and essential nutrients can lead to overall digestive imbalances, making you more susceptible to food retention.

Beyond what's on your plate, your daily habits and internal balance play a crucial role. In TCM, Qi represents your vital energy. If your digestive Qi is weak — perhaps due to stress, overwork, or a weakened Spleen and Stomach — your system simply lacks the power to process food effectively.

Dampness and phlegm accumulation are TCM concepts referring to an excess of fluids and metabolic waste. When these build up, they can physically obstruct your digestive system, acting like a literal clog. Similarly, if the flow of Qi and Blood in your digestive organs becomes blocked or stagnant, it directly interferes with digestion, causing food to stagnate in your gut.

Your emotions also have a direct impact on your digestion; stress or excessive worry can significantly affect the Spleen and Stomach, leading to digestive disturbances. Finally, a sedentary lifestyle slows down everything, including your digestion. Regular movement helps keep your digestive system active and efficient. Understanding these underlying causes in TCM can empower you to make more informed choices about your diet and lifestyle to prevent and address food retention.

How Food Retention Can Affect Our Body

In Traditional Chinese Medicine, food retention isn't just about a full stomach; it can have a wide range of negative effects on your body. When undigested food lingers in your digestive system, it disrupts the harmonious flow of your body's vital systems.

One of the primary consequences of food retention is the formation of dampness and phlegm. In TCM, dampness is considered heavy, cloudy, and sticky, while phlegm is thick and obstructive. These unwelcome substances can impede the flow of Qi and Blood throughout your body, leading to a variety of health complaints.

Naturally, the most immediate impact is digestive discomfort. You might experience bloating, a feeling of fullness, abdominal distension, and general unease. These symptoms can be quite disruptive to your daily life. Food retention also frequently leads to irregular bowel movements, ranging from constipation to diarrhea, or even alternating bouts of both. Stools may become loose, foul-smelling, or difficult to pass.

Beyond digestive issues, the accumulation of dampness and phlegm can manifest as fatigue and a sense of heaviness. You might feel perpetually tired, lacking in energy, and experience heavy limbs. Critically, when food isn't properly digested and absorbed, your body struggles to get the nutrients it needs, potentially leading to reduced nutrient absorption and deficiencies in vital substances like Qi and Blood. In some cases, this accumulation can even contribute to weight gain due to excess fluid retention and fat storage.

TCM emphasizes the interconnectedness of the body. Food retention can directly impact the Spleen and Stomach, the organs crucial for digestion and transformation. This disruption can then cascade, affecting other organ systems and leading to widespread imbalances. Furthermore, the digestive system is closely linked to emotional well-being. Food retention can contribute to emotional disturbances such as irritability, mood swings, and, in some instances, even depression. If left unaddressed, chronic food retention can contribute to more serious chronic health conditions over time, including persistent digestive disorders, obesity, metabolic imbalances, and even respiratory issues linked to dampness and phlegm accumulation.

Different Individuals May Experience Different Symptoms With Multiple Dark To Light Watery Stools Within A Day

Abdominal Discomfort. Patients may experience abdominal fullness, bloating, distension, or discomfort. This sensation is often described as feeling overly full, even if they haven't eaten.

Nausea and Vomiting. Nausea and occasional vomiting can occur, especially if there is significant stagnation of undigested food.

Belching. Frequent belching or burping is a common symptom of food retention. The belch may have a foul or sour odor, indicative of undigested food after a large meal.

Acid Reflux. Patients may experience acid reflux or heartburn due to the pressure of undigested food pushing back into the esophagus.

Bad Breath. Foul breath, often described as a "rotten" or unpleasant odor, can result from the fermentation of undigested food in the stomach.

Lack of Appetite. Food retention can lead to a reduced or suppressed appetite, as the person may still feel full from a previous meal.

Constipation or Diarrhea. Stool irregularities can occur. Some individuals may experience constipation, while others may have loose stools or diarrhea.

Fatigue and Heaviness. Patients often report feeling tired and sluggish, as if their energy is weighed down by the undigested food.

Taste Changes. There may be a lingering unpleasant taste in the mouth, often described as bitter or sour.

Coated Tongue. The tongue may have a thick, greasy coating, which is a common diagnostic sign in TCM for food retention.

Self-Care and Support

Rest and Hydrate. Rest is essential to allow the body to recover. Focus on staying hydrated by drinking clear fluids like water, herbal teas, or clear broths to prevent dehydration caused by vomiting or diarrhea.

Begin With a Bland Diet. Choose easily digestible foods like congee (rice porridge) or plain rice, which are gentle on the stomach.

Reduce Portion Size. Eat smaller, more frequent meals to ease the digestive process.

Apply Acupressure. Certain acupressure points, such as PC-6 (Neiguan) and ST-36 (Zusanli), may be massaged to relieve nausea and vomiting.

Consult a TCM Practitioner. If symptoms are severe, prolonged, or accompanied by other concerning signs, consult a qualified TCM practitioner for a personalized assessment and treatment plan.

Foods To Relieve Food Retention

Mung bean. Mung beans are sometimes used for their cooling properties and are considered beneficial for detoxification and balancing the body's energies. It is best for dark watery stools with a foul smell.

Ginger. Ginger is well-known for its digestive benefits. It can help alleviate symptoms of food retention. Consider drinking a small amount ginger tea or adding fresh ginger to your meals. Ginger is warming, so it is best when the diarrhea is light yellow to clear.

Mint. Peppermint or spearmint tea can have a soothing effect on the stomach and promote digestion. Because mint is slightly cooling in nature, it is best to drink when the watery stool still has some brown color.

Rice congee (porridge). Rice congee is a staple in TCM for addressing digestive issues. It's gentle on the stomach and can help clear food stagnation. You can add mild seasonings like a pinch of salt or a drizzle of sesame oil.

Steamed or boiled vegetables. Steamed or boiled vegetables like bok choy, Chinese cabbage, or zucchini are easy to digest and can be beneficial for relieving food retention.

Cooked grains. Opt for well-cooked grains like rice, oats, or millet instead of heavy, hard-to-digest grains like brown rice or quinoa.

Bananas. Bananas are considered easy to digest and can be a good choice if you're experiencing digestive discomfort.

Papaya. Papaya contains enzymes like papain that aid digestion. It can be eaten fresh but not in cold smoothies.

Warm water. Sip warm water throughout the day to help clear food stagnation and promote digestive flow.

Rice vinegar. A very small amount of rice vinegar, diluted in water, can be sipped before or after meals to support digestion.

Herbs. Herbs to clear Food Stagnation, expel toxins, and regulate digestion include Hawthorn Fruit (Shan Zha), Raphanus Seed (Lai Fu Zi), Forsythia Fruit (Lian Qiao), and Coptis Root (Huang Lian). It is best to work with a qualified TCM practitioner when using herbal formulas. For daily support, herbal teas such as chrysanthemum tea or hawthorn tea may be beneficial for digestion. These can be consumed warm or at room temperature.

Fennel seeds. Chewing on a few fennel seeds after meals can help ease digestion and reduce bloating.

Lemon water. A glass of warm lemon water in the morning is often recommended to stimulate digestion and gently awaken the system. In TCM, lemon is considered warm in nature and sour in flavor, which can help promote digestion and move stagnation when used in moderation and suited to an individual's constitution. However, taken daily on an empty stomach — especially for those with chronic digestive issues — lemon water may irritate the Stomach lining or further weaken digestive fire over time.

Bone broth. If you consume meat, homemade bone broth can be soothing and nutritious for the digestive system.

Aloe vera juice. A small amount of aloe vera juice, preferably without added sugars, can help soothe the stomach lining. Keep in mind that aloe vera is a very cold medicinal. It is best when there is an excess of heat in the digestive system (when stools are foul smelling).

Foods That Can Worsen Food Retention

Fried and greasy foods. Foods that are deep-fried or cooked with excessive oil can be challenging to digest and may contribute to food retention.

Spicy foods. Spices and seasonings that are overly spicy or hot may irritate the digestive system and worsen food retention.

Raw foods. While raw fruits and vegetables have many health benefits, they can be harder to digest for some individuals, especially if they have a weakened digestive system.

Processed foods. Highly processed and packaged foods often contain artificial additives, preservatives, and unhealthy fats, making them less digestible.

Large meals. Consuming overly large portions of food in one sitting can overwhelm the digestive system and lead to food retention.

Carbonated beverages. Carbonated drinks can introduce excess air into the digestive tract, potentially causing discomfort and bloating.

Dairy. Some people may have difficulty digesting dairy products, particularly if they are lactose intolerant.

Rich desserts. Very sweet or rich desserts can be taxing on the digestive system, especially after a heavy meal.

Alcohol. Excessive alcohol consumption can impair digestion and lead to discomfort and indigestion.

Caffeine. Coffee and other caffeinated beverages may stimulate acid production in the stomach, potentially worsening food retention in some individuals.

Over-the-counter medications. Be cautious with over-the-counter medications like antidiarrheal drugs, as they can sometimes trap toxins in the body.

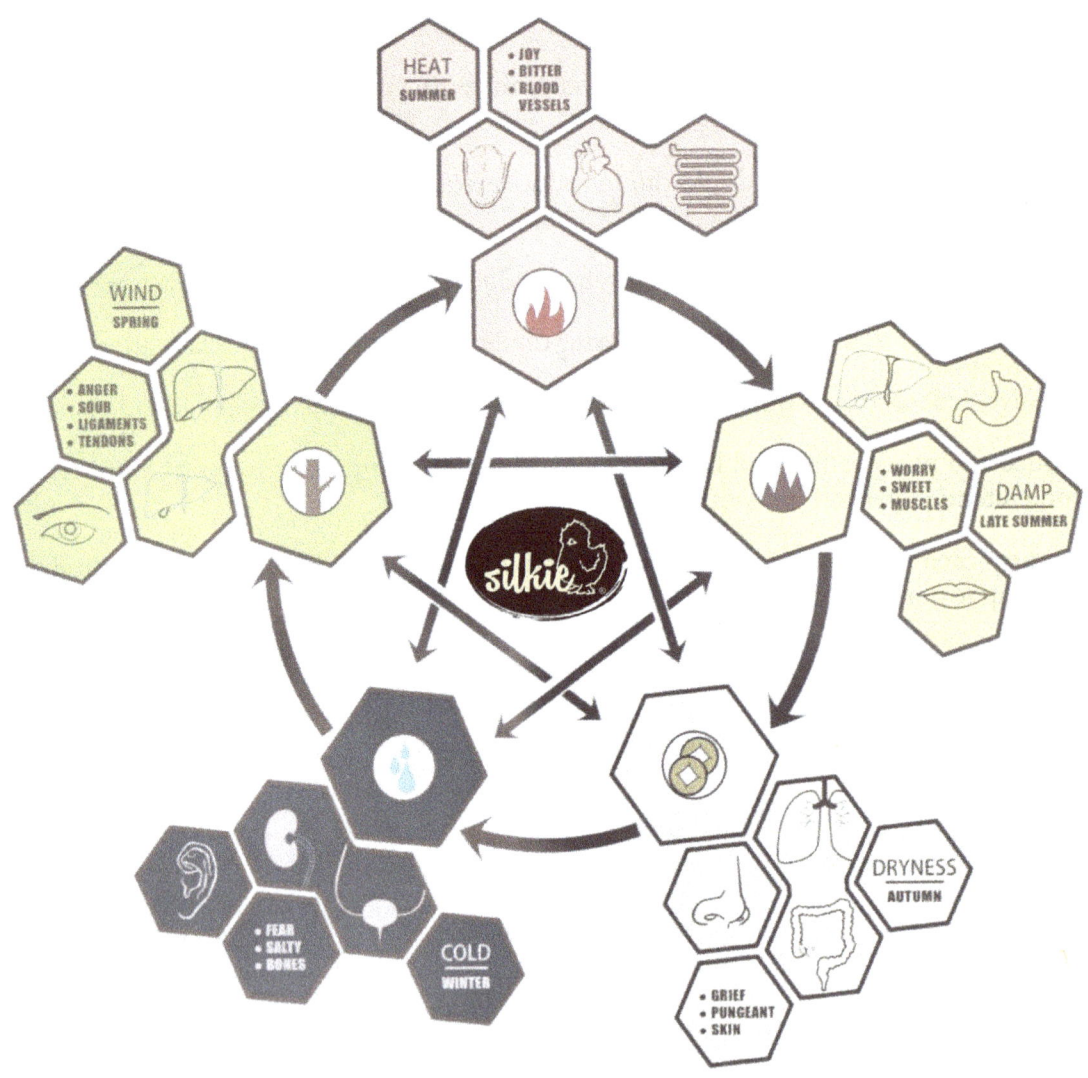

12. Dark Yellow, Watery Stool With or Without Foul Odor - Indicative of Heat and Dampness in the Stomach and Spleen

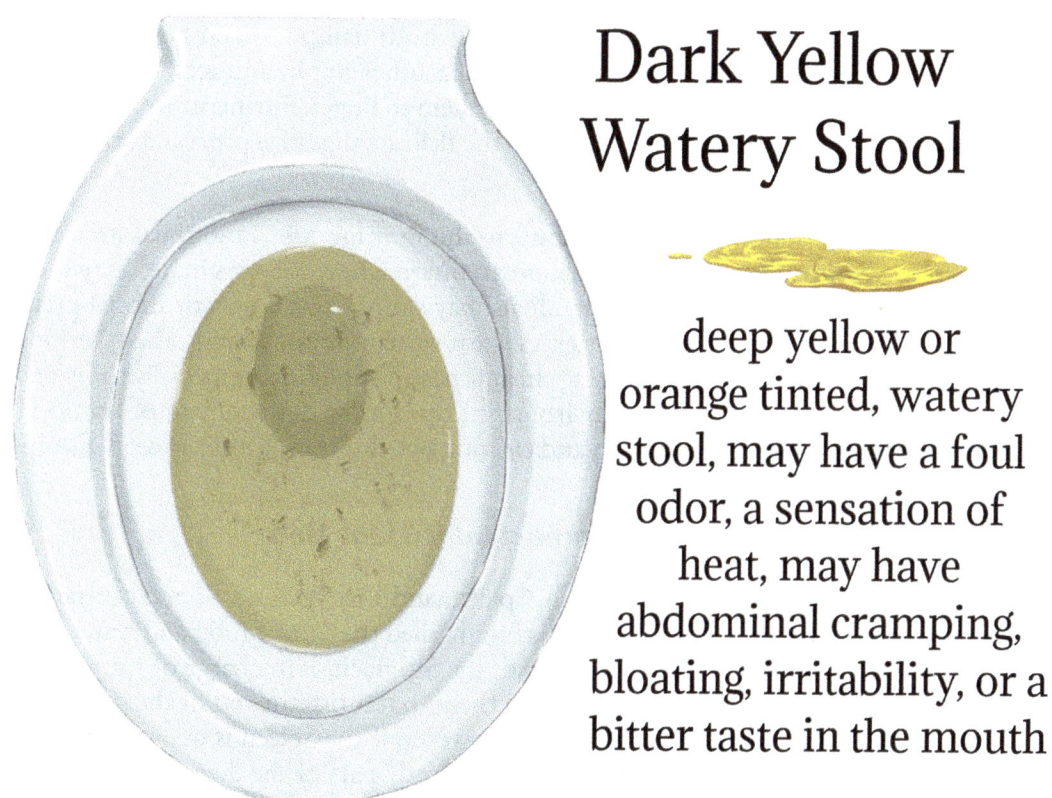

Dark Yellow Watery Stool

deep yellow or orange tinted, watery stool, may have a foul odor, a sensation of heat, may have abdominal cramping, bloating, irritability, or a bitter taste in the mouth

Figure 6.12 Darker yellow, watery stool, prolonged Liver and Spleen disharmony, Damp-Heat in the Intestines or Liver overacting on the Spleen.

What it Means: Dark yellow, watery stool that is stinky indicates excessive heat in your digestive system with dampness. Strong foul odor is almost always a pattern of Heat and Dampness. In Traditional Chinese Medicine, this pattern reflects an internal heat combined with dampness affecting the digestive organs. The Liver may become overheated and disrupt the Spleen's function of transforming and transporting food and fluids, leading to loose stool and excess moisture. The darker yellow or orange hue suggests heat pushing bile more rapidly through the intestines, giving the stool its tinted color. Individuals with dietary habits that include excessive consumption of spicy, greasy, or fried foods may be more prone to developing this condition. Individuals who feel hot or who have a lot of phlegm or mucus internally may also be prone to this condition.

Heat and Dampness in the Stomach and Spleen is a distinct condition and is not necessarily more severe than Spleen Yang Deficiency; rather, it represents a different pattern of imbalance. Here are the possible causes.

Underlying Causes

Ever experienced that uncomfortable feeling of being both overheated, sweaty and/or sluggish, especially after a rich meal? In Traditional Chinese Medicine, these sensations often point to a pattern known as Damp-Heat in the Stomach and Spleen. It's like having a sticky, hot mess brewing in your digestive core. Let's uncover the main culprits that can ignite this internal imbalance.

Our plates often hold the biggest clues. An abundance of spicy, greasy, and fried foods is a surefire way to fan the flames and introduce stickiness into your digestive system. Think of them as contributing to a stagnant, hot environment. Similarly, indulging in rich, fatty foods in excess, or going overboard on sugary and sweet treats, can create conditions where both heat and dampness flourish. And don't forget your beverages! Excessive alcohol and caffeine are notorious for generating internal heat, which then often combines with dampness to create this uncomfortable pattern.

Beyond what we consume, our environment and daily routines also play a significant role. Living in hot and humid climates can make us more susceptible to accumulating both dampness and heat, as our bodies absorb these qualities from our surroundings. A sedentary lifestyle and insufficient physical activity also hinder the body's natural ability to disperse excess heat and dampness, allowing them to linger. Furthermore, irregular eating habits — like skipping meals or eating too quickly — can disrupt the delicate digestive process, further contributing to dampness.

Even our inner world and underlying health can contribute to this fiery muddle. Emotional stress and imbalances, particularly unresolved anger or frustration, can contribute to internal heat patterns in TCM, which then readily combine with any pre-existing dampness. Some individuals may simply have a constitutional predisposition — a natural tendency — towards accumulating either excess heat or dampness, making them more prone to this challenging pattern from the get-go. Finally, underlying chronic health conditions, especially those that persistently affect the digestive system, can over time create an environment ripe for the development of Damp-Heat patterns. Understanding these triggers is key to cooling down and clearing out this unwelcome internal Damp-Heat.

Why The Stomach, Spleen and Liver Are Important To Our Body

In Traditional Chinese Medicine (TCM), the Stomach, Spleen, and Liver are considered central to maintaining health and balance throughout the body. The Stomach is often called the "sea of food and water," responsible for receiving and breaking down food. The Spleen, paired with the Stomach, is in charge of transforming that food into Qi (energy), Blood, and body fluids, then transporting them to nourish the rest of the body. A strong Spleen ensures proper digestion, a clear mind, and steady energy. However, if the Spleen is weak, it can lead to bloating, fatigue, loose stools, and poor appetite. The Liver, while not directly part of the digestive process, plays a crucial role in regulating the smooth flow of Qi throughout the body, including digestive Qi. When Liver Qi is flowing smoothly, emotions are stable, digestion is efficient, and the body feels balanced.

Liver Qi Stagnation occurs when the flow of Liver energy becomes blocked or constrained, often due to emotional stress, frustration, or lack of movement. In TCM, this can manifest physically as bloating, belching, indigestion, constipation, or alternating constipation and diarrhea. Emotionally, it can lead to mood swings, irritability, depression, or a feeling of being "stuck." Since the Liver supports the Spleen's function, when Liver Qi is stagnant, it can overact on the Spleen and disrupt digestion — creating symptoms like gas, nausea, and irregular bowel movements. Releasing Liver Qi and supporting its smooth flow through gentle movement, emotional expression, proper rest, and herbal support is essential to restore harmony in the body.

Different Individuals May Experience Different Symptoms With Darker Yellow, Watery Stool And a Foul "Stinky" Odor

Digestive Issues. Heat and dampness in the Stomach and Spleen often leads to digestive problems like foul-smelling diarrhea, abdominal pain and discomfort, especially after eating, nausea and vomiting, and feeling of fullness and bloating in the abdomen

Thirst. Excessive heat in the digestive system can lead to increased thirst and a preference for cold drinks.

Appetite Changes. There may be a reduced or variable appetite, with cravings for cold and refreshing foods and drinks.

Heaviness. People with this pattern may feel heavy, lethargic, and sluggish in their body and mind.

Fatigue. Chronic fatigue and a lack of energy are common, as the body's digestive system is working inefficiently.

Swelling. Heat and Dampness can cause edema or swelling, particularly in the lower extremities.

Urine Changes. There may be dark, concentrated urine, which can be strong-smelling.

Tongue and Pulse. TCM practitioners often examine the tongue and pulse to diagnose patterns. In a heat and dampness pattern, the tongue may have a thick, greasy, yellow coating, and the pulse may be slippery or rapid.

Skin Issues. Excess heat and dampness can sometimes manifest as skin problems, such as acne, rashes, or eczema.

Emotional Factors. This pattern may also affect emotions. Heat can make a person irritable, agitated, and easily angered.

Self-Care and Support

Manage Stress. Emotional stress can contribute to heat accumulation. Engage in relaxation techniques like meditation, tai chi, or yoga.

Exercise. Engage in regular, gentle exercise to promote circulation and support overall health.

Avoid Overexertion. Excessive physical exertion can worsen dampness and heat conditions. Strike a balance between activity and rest.

Herbal Remedies. Consult with a TCM practitioner for herbal formulas tailored to your specific condition. Herbal like Scutellaria (Huang Qin), Coptis (Huang Lian), and Alisma (Ze Xie) can help clear heat, resolve dampness, and harmonize the Stomach and Spleen.

Acupuncture. Acupuncture with a qualified TCM practitioner can help rebalance the body's energy, clear heat, and address dampness.

Mindful Eating. Eat slowly and mindfully to aid digestion. Avoid overeating or consuming heavy meals close to bedtime.

Rest and Sleep. Ensure you get adequate rest and quality sleep, as this supports the body's natural healing processes.

Avoid Damp Environments. Minimize exposure to damp or humid environments, as these can exacerbate dampness-related symptoms.

Regular TCM Consultations. Consult regularly with a qualified TCM practitioner who can assess your progress and adjust treatment as needed.

Foods To Relieve Heat And Dampness In The Stomach And Spleen

Below are foods that have a cooling nature to counteract heat and dampness:

Bitter foods can help clear heat and reduce dampness. Examples include bitter gourd, bitter melon, dandelion greens, and bitter herbs like gentian root and should be consumed in moderation to avoid over cooling the system and creating potential digestive issues like diarrhea.

Fruits with a cooling nature can help reduce heat and dampness. Consider including water-rich fruits like watermelon, cantaloupe, cucumber, and citrus fruits in your diet and should be consumed in moderation.

Leafy greens, like lettuce, spinach, and kale, are cooling and can help clear heat and dampness.

Mung beans are known for their ability to clear heat and dampness. They can be used in soups, porridge, or as a base for desserts, and should be consumed in moderation.

Whole grains, like brown rice and oats can help nourish the Spleen and support healthy digestion. While some grains — such as millet or coix seed — are especially useful for reducing Dampness, others should be consumed in moderation if Damp accumulation is present. Choosing the right grains for your body type and preparing them well (cooked, warm, and simple) can help maintain digestive balance.

Lean proteins, like skinless poultry, fish, and tofu, are not excessively hot in nature and can be added into your meals without exacerbating heat conditions. For example, tofu is cooling and can be used in various dishes to balance the heat.

Herbs to clear Heat, drain Dampness, and harmonize the digestive organs include Scutellaria Root (Huang Qin), Phellodendron Bark (Huang Bai), Alisma (Ze Xie), and Gardenia Fruit (Zhi Zi). It is best to work with a qualified TCM practitioner when using herbal formulas. For daily support, herbal teas made from cooling herbs like chrysanthemum, mint, and lotus leaf can be beneficial.

Porridge or congee can be soothing to the digestive system and is easily digestible.

Water and diluted fruit juices help with hydration. Water also helps to flush out excess Heat and Dampness. Herbal teas and diluted fruit juices can also be hydrating.

Foods That Can Worsen Heat And Dampness In The Stomach And Spleen

Spicy foods, like chili peppers, hot sauces, and excessive use of spices like ginger and garlic, can increase heat and dampness in the body. These foods may irritate the digestive system and lead to more pronounced symptoms.

Greasy and fried foods, like fast food, fried chicken, and French fries, can contribute to dampness and heat. They are often high in unhealthy fats and can be difficult to digest.

Dairy products, like milk, cheese, and butter can create dampness and mucus in the digestive system for some individuals, exacerbating the condition.

Overconsumption of sweets, like candies, desserts, and cookies, can lead to increased dampness and heat. These foods may disrupt the balance of blood sugar levels and contribute to heat-related symptoms.

Alcohol tends to be hot and damp in nature. In excess, alcohol can worsen symptoms of heat and dampness.

Processed and refined foods, including white bread, sugary cereals, and processed snacks, are often devoid of nutrients and can create imbalances in the digestive system.

Overconsumption of meat, especially red meat, and fatty cuts, can be heating and may contribute to dampness. Moderation is key when including meat in the diet.

High-sodium meals can increase fluid retention and contribute to dampness in the body. Reducing salt intake can help manage dampness.

Cold and raw foods, while not necessarily heat-inducing, may weaken the digestive fire (Spleen Yang) and exacerbate dampness. Cooking or lightly steaming vegetables can make them easier to digest.

Heavy and rich foods that are difficult to digest, like creamy sauces and heavy gravies, can burden the digestive system and lead to dampness.

Caffeine from coffee, energy drinks, and certain teas can be heating and may disrupt digestion.

Sodas and carbonated drinks can introduce excess gas into the digestive system, potentially exacerbating bloating and discomfort associated with dampness.

13. Light Yellow, Watery Stool With or Without a Foul "Fishy" Odor - Indicative of Cold with Dampness in the Stomach and Spleen

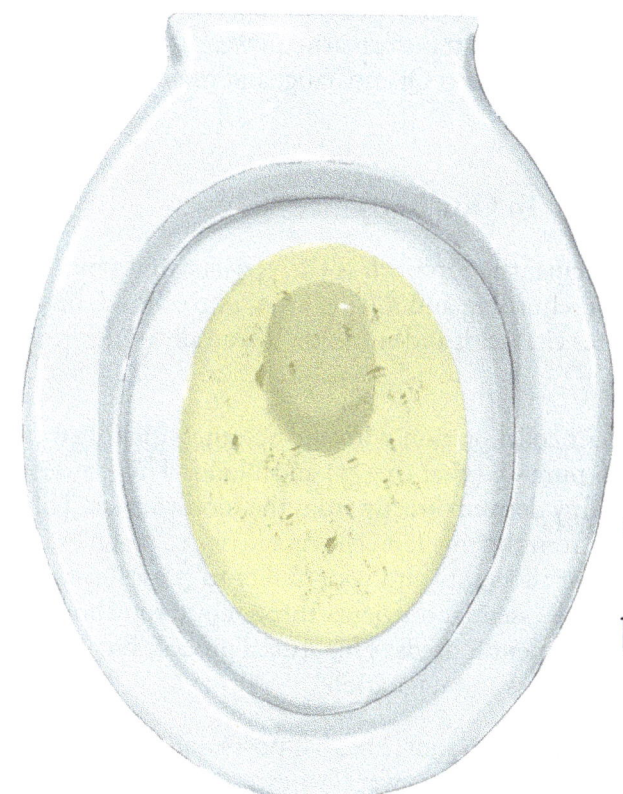

Light Yellow Watery Stool

pale yellow, watery stool, no solid pieces, mildly sour or foul odor, possible fatigue, cold hands and feet, bloating, low appetite, or a sensation of heaviness

Figure 6.13 Light yellowish watery poop, Chronic Deficiency of Spleen Qi, Spleen Yang Deficiency, Cold and Dampness in the Stomach and Spleen.

What It Means: Light yellow, watery stool with a foul odor that smells a bit fishy is a sign of excessive cold and dampness in your digestive system, more specifically in the Stomach and Spleen. Anyone can potentially have light yellow, watery stools from overeating cold or mucus-producing foods like dairy. In Traditional Chinese Medicine, the Spleen and Stomach are responsible for digesting food and transforming it into energy (Qi), Blood, and body fluids. When the Spleen's warming Yang energy is weak, its ability to transform and transport fluids fails, allowing excess moisture (Dampness) to build up. This results in a thin, watery stool that is light in color due to insufficient bile and poor digestive fire. Individuals who run cold or who have a lot of phlegm or mucus may be more prone to this type of yellow, watery stool.

When you habitually consume dairy, fatty, greasy, sugary, or cold foods in excess, the Stomach and Spleen may become burdened with Cold and Dampness. It can lead to various digestive issues like abdominal discomfort, bloating, diarrhea, and a feeling of heaviness. Cold and Dampness in the Stomach and Spleen can be seen as a specific type of Spleen Yang Deficiency. While both conditions involve Spleen dysfunction, the presence of Cold and Dampness makes this condition more complex and may require specific dietary and lifestyle adjustments.

Underlying Causes

Light yellow watery stool in TCM often reflects a chronic deficiency of Spleen Qi and Spleen Yang, combined with an internal buildup of Cold and Dampness in the digestive system. The Spleen is responsible for transforming food into Qi and Blood and transporting fluids throughout the body. When Spleen Qi becomes weak over time —

due to poor diet, overthinking, irregular eating habits, or chronic illness — its ability to transform and transport weakens. As a result, fluids accumulate in the digestive tract, leading to unformed, loose, or watery stools. If this deficiency deteriorates into Spleen Yang Deficiency, the body's warming function also declines, allowing Cold to enter and further slow digestion. Cold impairs the Spleen's ability to "cook" and extract nutrients, while Dampness contributes to a feeling of heaviness, bloating, fatigue, and stool that lacks shape and consistency. The light yellow color of the stool indicates a weak digestive fire rather than a heat condition. Together, this pattern suggests a long-standing internal Cold-Damp condition due to weakened transformative power of the Spleen and Stomach. Addressing this requires warming the abdomen, tonifying Spleen Qi and Yang, and resolving internal Dampness through appropriate diet, herbs, and lifestyle adjustments.

Why The Stomach and Spleen Are Important To Our Body

In the intricate world of Traditional Chinese Medicine, the Stomach is the very starting point of our body's nourishment. Imagine it as a powerful digesting pot, churning and mixing every bite of food, breaking it down into smaller, more manageable particles. It also secretes vital acids and enzymes, chemically transforming your meal to prepare it for its next journey.

But the Stomach doesn't work alone. It's in constant collaboration with the Spleen, which then takes over the crucial role of transforming that digested food into pure Qi (vital energy) and Blood. This powerful duo is the engine that generates your "postnatal Qi" — the energy derived directly from the food you eat. This Qi isn't just for movement; it fuels every single bodily function, from the smallest cellular activity to the grand operations of your organs and musculoskeletal system, ensuring overall vitality and your ability to resist illness. The Stomach and Spleen also work hand-in-hand to distribute these essential nutrients throughout your body, guaranteeing that every organ, muscle, and tissue receives the nourishment it needs. This crucial process also involves managing fluids, preventing the uncomfortable build-up of dampness and stagnation.

The Spleen plays a significant role in immune function. As the source of that postnatal Qi, the Spleen powers all your body's defenses, including your immune system, helping you ward off external pathogens. While Western medicine might focus on white blood cells and antibodies, TCM sees the Spleen as the vital fuel station that keeps your immunity strong.

Beyond the physical, your digestive well-being is deeply connected to your mental and emotional health. In TCM, a healthy Stomach and Spleen are vital for clear thinking, emotional stability, and a general sense of well-being. Think of phrases like "chew the fat," "mull it over," or "ruminate" – they all reflect this ancient understanding that how we process our food directly impacts how we process our thoughts and feelings.

These digestive powerhouses — the Stomach and Spleen — also play a role in regulating your body's internal temperature, helping to maintain a harmonious, balanced warmth. In TCM, Spleen Yang serves as a key source of internal warmth in the body, so healthy digestion — through the combined efforts of the Spleen and Stomach — not only transforms food into energy but also helps regulate body temperature. They are also deeply connected to weight management. When food is fully digested and efficiently transformed into usable Qi and Blood, the body feels genuinely nourished, reducing unnecessary cravings and the tendency to overeat. Moreover, strong digestion helps prevent the accumulation of 'phlegm' or 'mucus' — residual byproducts of incomplete digestion — which can manifest as bloating, water retention, and unwanted weight gain.

Ultimately, the Stomach and Spleen are central to TCM's holistic view of health. Their proper functioning influences nearly every aspect of your well-being, highlighting the intricate interconnectedness of body, mind, and emotions.

Different Individuals May Experience Different Symptoms With Light Yellow, Watery Stool With a Foul "Fishy" Odor

Abdominal Distension. This condition can be accompanied by abdominal pain, audible stomach rumbling (borborygmus), or a feeling of fullness in the upper abdomen (epigastric distension). Individuals often experience a sense of fullness, bloating, or discomfort in the abdominal area. There may also be a feeling of heaviness.

Diarrhea. Food and drinks that are cold and damp in nature easily weaken the digestive fire, which can lead to loose or watery stools. Diarrhea may be chronic or intermittent.

Fatigue. Cold and dampness can sap energy and lead to a general feeling of tiredness or lethargy. Individuals may lack vitality and motivation.

Nausea. Some individuals may experience nausea or queasiness, especially after eating cold or raw foods.

Loss of Appetite. Cold and damp conditions can lead to a reduced appetite, making it difficult for individuals to eat a sufficient amount of food.

Taste Changes. There may be alterations in taste perception, often described as a "bland" or "lack of taste" sensation in the mouth.

Thick and Sticky Tongue Coating. On examination of the tongue, a TCM practitioner may observe a white and sticky coating, which is indicative of dampness.

Feeling of Coldness. Individuals with cold and dampness may feel excessively cold, even in warm environments. With Yang Deficiency, you may be very sensitive to cold, air conditioning, or drafts. Cold sensitivity may be accompanied by a mild fever, headache, and nasal congestion. Typically there is a preference for warm or hot beverages and foods.

Joint and Muscle Pain. Dampness can accumulate in the joints and muscles, leading to discomfort, stiffness, aches, and pain. These symptoms tend to be worse in damp or cold weather.

Heaviness. There is often a sensation of heaviness throughout the body, which can affect mobility and overall comfort.

Difficulty Concentrating. Mental fog, difficulty concentrating, and a sense of mental sluggishness may be present, impacting cognitive function.

Sensitivity to Humidity. Individuals with cold and dampness may be particularly sensitive to humid weather, which can exacerbate symptoms.

Self-Care and Support

Dietary Modifications. Adjust your diet to favor foods that are warm and strengthen the Spleen and Stomach. Avoid cold, mucus-producing foods like cold beverages, dairy, raw foods, and excessive sweets. Include warm, cooked meals with an emphasis on easily digestible foods. Add ginger, garlic, cinnamon, and other warming spices to your cooked vegetables.

Balanced Eating Habits. Establish regular eating patterns with three meals a day at consistent times. Avoid overeating or undereating. Chew your food thoroughly to aid digestion.

Warm Foods and Beverages. Opt for warm or room temperature foods and drinks.

Cooking Methods. Use cooking methods like steaming, stewing, or stir-frying, which retain warmth and are more suitable for individuals with cold and damp patterns.

Hydration. Stay adequately hydrated with warm or room temperature water. Sip on herbal teas with ginger, cinnamon, fennel, or cardamom can be soothing and warming for the digestion system.

Gentle Movement. Engage in gentle exercises like tai chi or Qigong to promote circulation and warmth in the body. Avoid excessive sweating or strenuous workouts that may exacerbate dampness. The pores have to open to release sweat. When the pores open, dampness can easily enter the body.

Warmth and Protection. Keep your abdomen and lower back warm, especially during cold weather. Consider using heating pads or warm compresses. Moxa heating packs made with mugwort are especially beneficial for Yang Deficiency with cold and dampness.

Stress Management. Stress can exacerbate TCM imbalances. Practice relaxation techniques like meditation, deep breathing, or yoga to reduce stress.

Rest and Sleep. Ensure you get adequate rest and quality sleep. TCM places great importance on the body's ability to replenish and restore during sleep.

Avoid Damp Environments. If possible, avoid damp and cold environments, as they can worsen your condition.

Consult a TCM Practitioner. For personalized guidance and treatment, consult with a TCM practitioner who can perform a thorough assessment of your condition and create an individualized treatment plan. Acupuncture treatments and herbal remedies can be tailored to your specific pattern of cold and dampness.

Foods To Relieve Cold And Dampness In The Stomach And Spleen

Warming foods. Focus on eating warm foods to counteract the cold and dampness. When cooking vegetables, add ginger, garlic, cinnamon, onions, or cloves to offset the cooling nature of leafy, green vegetables.

Cooked foods. Opt for cooked foods over raw foods. Cooking helps break down the cold nature of certain ingredients and aids digestion. Steamed or lightly stir-fried vegetables and well-cooked grains are suitable choices.

Root vegetables. Root vegetables like sweet potatoes, carrots, and butternut squash are warming and nourishing for the Spleen and Stomach. Include them in your meals.

Whole grains. Choose whole grains such as brown rice, quinoa, and oats. These grains are nourishing and easier to digest compared to refined grains.

Lean proteins. Incorporate lean sources of protein like chicken, turkey, lean cuts of beef, and tofu. These proteins support the Spleen and Stomach function without contributing to dampness.

Spices. Use warming spices like black pepper, cardamom, and cumin in your cooking to promote warmth and improve digestion.

Herbs. Herbs to warm the Spleen, dispel Cold, and dry Dampness include Dried Ginger (Gan Jiang), Atractylodes Rhizome (Cang Zhu), Poria (Fu Ling), and Magnolia Bark (Hou Po). It is best to work with a qualified TCM practitioner when using herbal formulas. For daily support, herbal teas made from warming herbs like cinnamon, ginger, and licorice can be soothing and beneficial for this pattern. Enjoy them between meals. Ginger tea is particularly helpful for cold and dampness in the Stomach and Spleen.

Moderate consumption. Avoid excessive consumption of dairy, as it can contribute to dampness. Limit sugary and sweet foods, which can also generate mucus and phlegm.

Bland foods. In TCM, bland foods like rice congee are often recommended for digestive comfort. Congee is a rice porridge that can be customized with various ingredients.

Bone broth. Homemade bone broth is nutritious and gentle on the digestive system. It can help strengthen the Spleen and Stomach.

Warm water. Drink warm or room temperature water throughout the day. Avoid iced or very cold drinks.

Balanced meals. Create balanced meals with a combination of carbohydrates, proteins, and vegetables. This supports overall digestive health.

Chew thoroughly. Practice mindful eating and chew your food thoroughly to aid digestion.

Foods That Can Worsen Cold And Dampness In The Stomach And Spleen

Cold drinks, especially those with ice, are considered harsh on the digestive system. They can weaken the digestive fire of the Stomach and hinder its ability to process food effectively.

Raw foods, such as salads, raw veggies and sushi, are typically considered cold in nature. They may be difficult to digest for individuals with Cold in the Stomach and Spleen.

Dairy products, including milk, yogurt, and cheese, are considered cold and mucus forming in TCM. It can lead to digestive issues for some individuals.

Coffee and caffeinated beverages are natural diuretics, which means they increase fluid loss. From a TCM perspective, this makes them especially unsuitable for people with light yellow watery stools, as the body is already losing fluids and further dehydration can weaken digestion and Qi.

Cucumbers are refreshing, therefore they are also cooling in nature. Excessive consumption of cucumbers can intensify cold in the Stomach and Spleen.

Watermelon is a hydrating fruit, but its cooling nature can be too much for people with digestive weakness.

Cold-pressed juices made from raw fruits and vegetables can be cold and may not sit well with those who have colds in the Stomach and Spleen.

Mint is a cooling herb often used in teas and desserts. It can have a chilling effect on the digestive system.

Ice cream is both cold and mucus-producing in TCM, which can contribute to digestive discomfort.

Frozen snacks can be overly cold and difficult to digest.

Raw fruits are healthy, but consuming large quantities of fruit, especially banana, melon, dragonfruit, and pear can be too cool for some individuals.

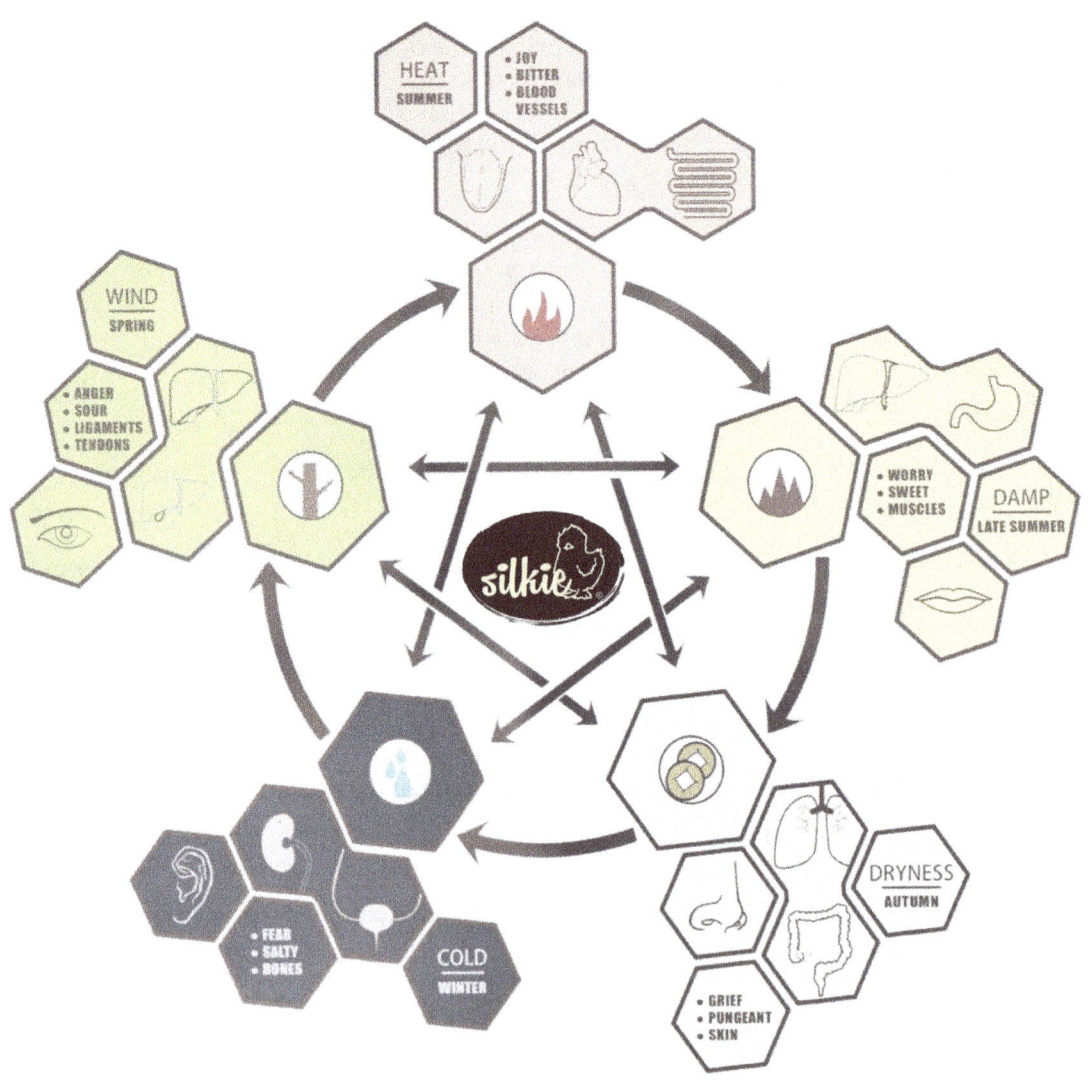

14. Green Stool – Sign of Liver Qi Stagnation with Damp-Heat in the Intestines

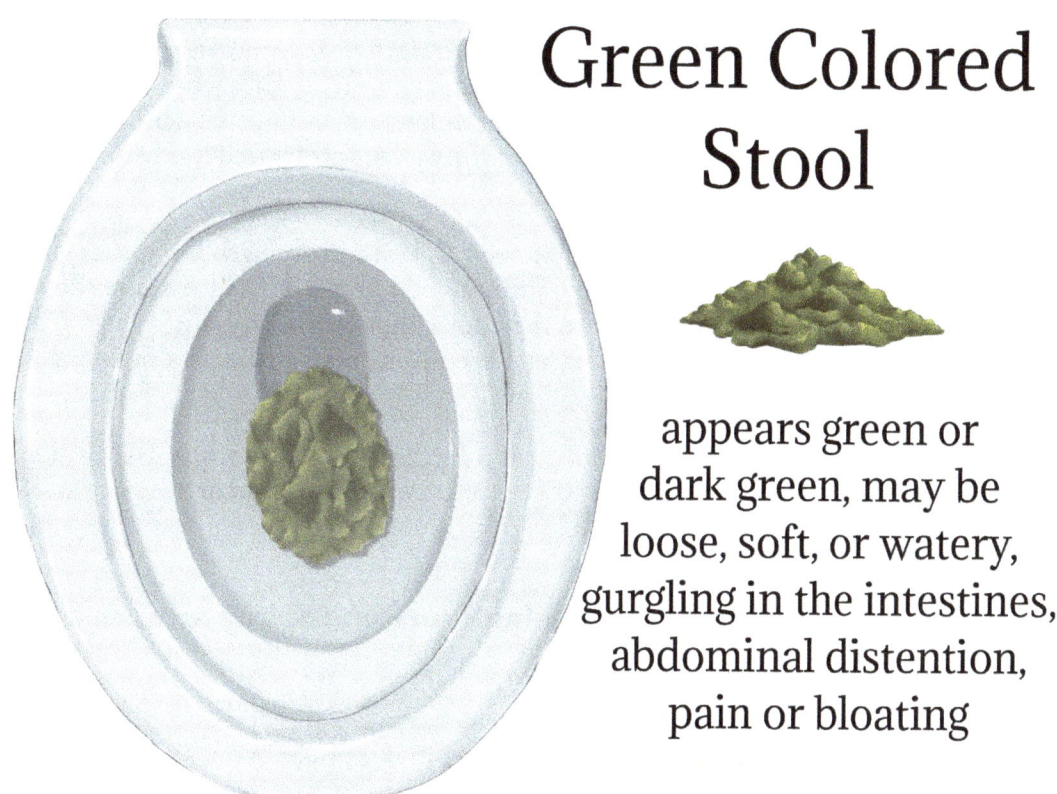

Green Colored Stool

appears green or dark green, may be loose, soft, or watery, gurgling in the intestines, abdominal distention, pain or bloating

Figure 6.14 Green stool, too much bile, Liver Qi Stagnation, Damp-Heat in the Intestines, or Spleen and Stomach Deficiency with Coldness.

What it Means: In Traditional Chinese Medicine, green stools often point toward a disharmony involving the Liver and Gallbladder, most commonly Liver Qi stagnation combined with Damp-Heat. The Liver governs the smooth flow of Qi throughout the body and works closely with the Gallbladder to store and excrete bile. When Liver Qi becomes stagnant — often from emotional stress, frustration, or unresolved anger — heat can build up in the Liver. If this heat combines with Dampness, bile may be released too quickly or excessively into the intestines, tinting the stool green. This pattern is often accompanied by abdominal discomfort, urgent or loose stools, mild irritability, and sometimes a bitter taste in the mouth.

Not all green stools are due to high concentration of bile. Sometimes, the color simply comes from eating a lot of leafy greens like spinach or kale, or from artificial food coloring in candies and drinks. However, If green stool is accompanied by diarrhea and pain in the lower right abdomen, more serious conditions such as intestinal inflammation or tumors could be involved.

Underlying Causes

From a TCM perspective, green stool can stem from three main patterns: Liver Qi stagnation, Damp-Heat in the Intestines, and Spleen and Stomach Deficiency with Coldness.

It often begins with disrupted Liver function, most commonly from emotional stress. When frustration, resentment, or ongoing pressure are not expressed or resolved, Liver Qi becomes stagnant. This stagnation not only disrupts the smooth flow of Qi but also affects the Liver's role in regulating bile secretion. Stagnant Liver Qi can generate internal Heat, which in turn disturbs the Gallbladder. Since bile is stored in the Gallbladder and released into the intestines to aid digestion, excessive or irregular bile secretion can alter stool color, often turning it green.

Damp-Heat in the Intestines is another key cause. This pattern develops when Dampness — caused by overeating greasy, fried, or heavily spiced foods — combines with Heat, often aggravated by alcohol or processed food intake. The Dampness slows digestive transformation, while Heat accelerates intestinal movement. This imbalance pushes food through the digestive tract too quickly, preventing bile from being fully reabsorbed in the small intestine. As a result, more bile remains in the stool, creating a darker green hue. Environmental dampness, such as living in humid climates or spending long hours in poorly ventilated spaces, can further feed this pattern by weakening the Spleen's fluid-transforming ability.

In some cases, green stool may appear not from Heat, but from Spleen and Stomach Deficiency with Coldness. In this pattern, the body's digestive "fire" is too weak to transform food properly. Coldness slows down the digestive process, allowing food to stagnate and bile to remain in the stool without adequate transformation into the normal brown color. Here, the green tone is usually lighter, and symptoms may include abdominal coldness, lack of appetite, loose or watery stools, and fatigue.

By identifying whether the root is Liver Qi Stagnation, Damp-Heat, or Cold Deficiency, TCM tailors treatment to restore balance — moving Liver Qi, clearing Heat and Dampness when necessary, or warming and strengthening the Spleen and Stomach when Cold is the cause.

How Liver Qi Stagnation, Damp-Heat in the Intestines, and Spleen & Stomach Deficiency with Coldness Can Affect the Body

These three TCM patterns may all lead to green stool, but their effects go far beyond stool color. Liver Qi stagnation disrupts the smooth flow of energy, often triggered by emotional stress or frustration. This can cause mood swings, chest tightness, rib-side discomfort, and irregular bile release, which in turn impacts digestion.

Damp-Heat in the Intestines overloads the digestive system with pathological moisture and internal heat. The intestines may speed up transit time, pushing food through before bile can be fully reabsorbed. This not only alters stool color but can also cause bloating, foul-smelling stools, abdominal pain, and a sticky sensation in the mouth.

Spleen & Stomach Deficiency with Coldness weakens the body's digestive "fire," slowing the transformation of food into usable Qi and Blood. The result can be chronic fatigue, abdominal coldness, watery or loose stools, and a pale complexion. In this case, the green stool tends to be lighter, reflecting incomplete transformation of bile rather than excess bile secretion.

Different Individuals May Experience Different Symptoms With Green Colored Stool

Abdominal Discomfort. Mild cramping or pain in the upper right or middle abdomen is sometimes relieved after a bowel movement.

Urgent or Loose Stools. Some individuals may suddenly feel the need to defecate, often without much warning. The stool may be watery, soft, and occur more frequently than usual.

Bitter Taste in the Mouth. The unusual taste is linked to excess bile or Liver Heat and is especially noticeable in the morning.

Nausea or Reduced Appetite. Some individuals may have a feeling of queasiness or an aversion to rich, oily foods.

Bloating and Heaviness. Discomfort, particularly after meals, is due to Dampness obstructing digestion.

Irritability or Mood Swings. Emotional instability is linked to Liver Qi stagnation.

Tongue. Thick or thin yellowish coating often indicates Damp-Heat in the digestive system.

Restless Sleep. Problems with sleep include difficulty falling asleep or staying asleep and vivid dreaming.

Headaches or Eye Strain. Headaches on the sides of the head or behind the eyes reflect Liver and Gallbladder imbalance.

Dark or Strong-Smelling Urine. Darkness and strong odor are signs of internal Heat and concentrated bile excretion.

Mild Fever or Feeling of Warmth. Heat rising stems from the Damp-Heat pattern.

Fatigue. A combination of Qi stagnation and Dampness lead to low energy.

Skin Irritations. Rash, acne, or itching reflect internal Heat.

Self-Care and Support

Prioritize Emotional Well-Being. Practice stress-reduction methods such as meditation, journaling, or gentle breathing exercises to keep Liver Qi flowing.

Schedule Regular Physical Activity. Gentle stretching, yoga, Tai Chi, or walking can help move stagnant Qi and improve circulation.

Get Adequate Sleep. Aim to be in deep sleep during the Liver's peak time (11 PM to 3 AM) to support natural detoxification and bile production.

Avoid Overworking. Balance work and rest to prevent excess stress that can aggravate Liver Qi stagnation.

Manage Anger and Frustration. Express emotions in healthy ways and avoid prolonged emotional suppression.

Stay Hydrated. Drink warm or room-temperature water throughout the day to support smooth Qi and fluid movement.

Gentle Abdominal Massage. Light massage over the side of the ribs and upper abdomen can help relieve tension in the Liver area.

Foods to Relieve Liver Qi Stagnation with Damp-Heat in the Intestines

Lightly cooked green leafy vegetables. Spinach, bok choy, watercress, and dandelion greens help clear Liver Heat and promote smooth Qi flow.

Bitter vegetables. Bitter melon, kale, mustard greens, and romaine lettuce help drain Damp-Heat and support bile flow.

Cooling vegetables. Cucumber, celery, and zucchini help reduce Heat without harming digestion.

Herbs for cooking. Fresh mint, chrysanthemum flowers, and cilantro can help soothe the Liver and clear Heat.

Sprouted grains and legumes. Mung beans, adzuki beans, and barley help clear Dampness and support detoxification.

Whole grains. Brown rice, millet, and quinoa provide steady energy without creating Dampness.

Citrus peels and mildly sour foods. Tangerine peel in cooking, or small amounts of lemon or lime juice, help regulate Qi and aid digestion.

Mild spices. Turmeric and ginger in small amounts with the cooling green vegetables support digestion without adding Coldness or Heat.

White meats and light proteins. Steamed or boiled fish, chicken, or turkey provide nourishment without creating excess Damp-Heat.

Sea vegetables. Kelp, wakame, and nori soften stone-like hardness such as gallstones or masses that form from Damp-Heat in the Liver and Gallbladder. They also aid in clearing Heat and supporting healthy bile flow.

Herbs. Herbs to soothe the Intestines, regulate Qi, and clear Damp-Heat include Bupleurum Root (Chai Hu), Gentian Root (Long Dan Cao), Capillaris (Yin Chen Hao), and Alisma (Ze Xie). It is best to work with a qualified TCM practitioner when using herbal formulas. For daily support, herbal teas like Chrysanthemum tea, peppermint tea, or green tea (in moderation) to clear Heat and support Liver function.

Fruits (in moderation). Pears, apples, and watermelon cool Heat and hydrate. Fruits should be consumed at room temperature and not in excess.

Foods That Can Worsen Liver Qi Stagnation with Damp-Heat in the Intestines

Greasy, fried foods. Deep-fried snacks, fatty meats, and oily fast foods generate Damp-Heat and burden the Liver and Gallbladder.

Excessively spicy foods. Hot chili peppers, curry, and heavy seasoning can create internal Heat and irritate the digestive system.

Alcohol. Beer, wine, and spirits add both Dampness and Heat, overtaxing the Liver's detoxification function.

Excessive red meat. Lamb, beef, and other heavy meats are harder to digest and contribute to Damp-Heat formation.

Dairy products. Cheese, milk, cream, and ice cream produce Dampness, especially in those with weak digestion.

Processed and refined foods. Packaged snacks, refined sugars, and artificial additives disrupt Qi flow and produce Dampness.

Excessive sweets. Cakes, pastries, candy, and sugary drinks generate Dampness and stagnation.

Excessive nuts and seeds. While healthy in small amounts, overconsumption can create heaviness and contribute to Dampness.

Berries and citrus fruits. Their sour and warming nature can aggravate Liver Qi stagnation or Damp-Heat in the intestines.

Acidic foods. The sour flavor is astringent, which has the quality of holding and trapping Dampness-Heat, or toxins inside of the body. Damp-Heat needs to be drained and cleared from the body. Additionally, foods like vinegar, pickled vegetables, and citrus-heavy dressings — may irritate the Stomach and Liver in people already dealing with Damp-Heat, potentially worsening symptoms like bloating, nausea, or a bitter taste in the mouth.

Shellfish and rich seafood. Shrimp, crab, and lobster can be damp-producing and are best eaten sparingly.

Cold or iced drinks. Chilled beverages weaken digestion and slow Qi movement.

15. Pale Stool - Sign of Gallbladder or Liver issues

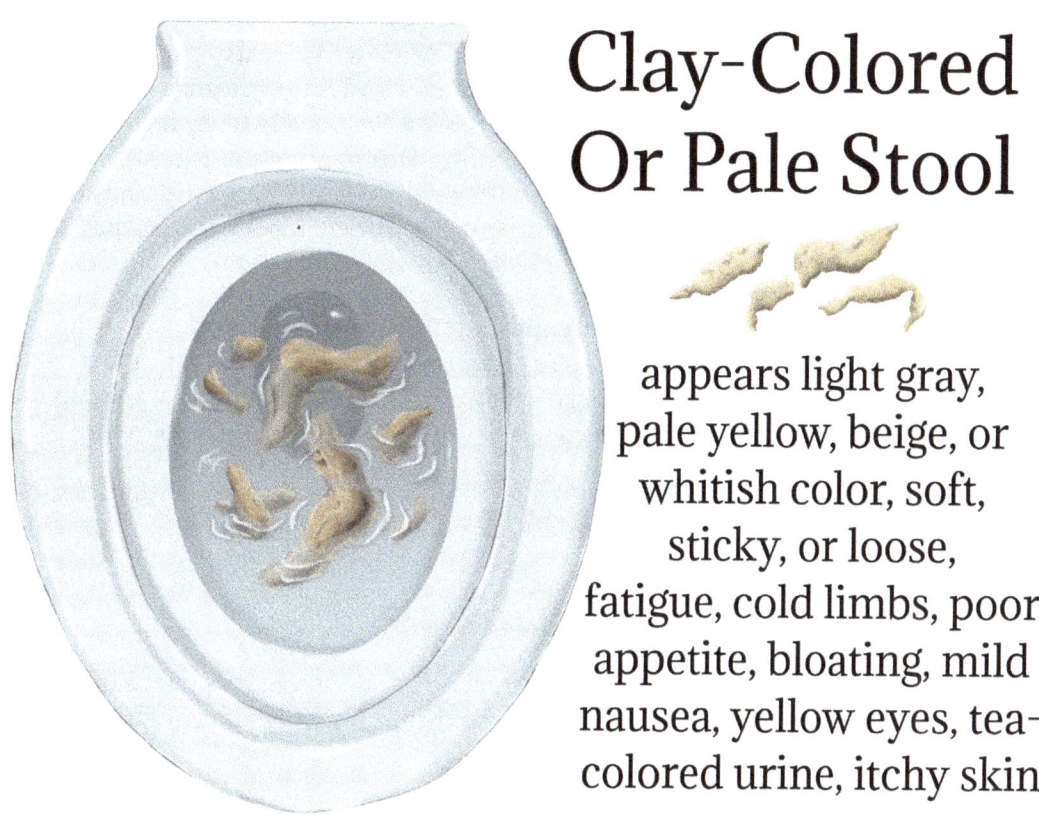

Clay-Colored Or Pale Stool appears light gray, pale yellow, beige, or whitish color, soft, sticky, or loose, fatigue, cold limbs, poor appetite, bloating, mild nausea, yellow eyes, tea-colored urine, itchy skin

Figure 6.15 Pale, gray, beige, whitish or clay-colored stool, Spleen Yang Deficiency, Liver Qi Stagnation, Gallbladder Damp-Heat, or Blood Deficiency.

What It Means: Has your stool ever appeared unusually pale or clay-colored? This striking change isn't just a random occurrence; it can be a significant red flag pointing to issues with your Liver or Gallbladder. In Traditional Chinese Medicine, pale or clay-colored stool typically reflects insufficient bile secretion, which is essential for giving stool its natural yellow-brown color. This can be caused by Damp-Heat obstructing the Gallbladder, Liver Qi not flowing smoothly, Blood Deficiency indirectly influencing stool color, or Spleen Yang Deficiency impairing transformation and transportation of fluids. This distinctive pale hue can be a telltale sign of conditions like gallstones, hepatitis, or cirrhosis, all of which require prompt medical attention.

Underlying Causes

In TCM, one of the primary causes of pale stools is a combination of Dampness and Spleen Yang Deficiency. Spleen Yang is your body's digestive engine, providing the warmth and energy needed to transform food into usable Qi, Blood, and nutrients. When Dampness builds up, it acts like a heavy fog, slowing and obstructing the Spleen's transformative power. Over time, this leads to inefficient digestion and the production of pale stools. Excessive intake of cold or raw foods can further weaken Spleen Yang, diminishing the digestive fire and impairing nutrient absorption, which also contributes to that pale, lackluster stool color.

Your Liver plays a crucial role in digestion, and its smooth functioning is vital for healthy stool color. In TCM, Liver Qi stagnation — often triggered by emotional stress, frustration, unresolved emotions, or lifestyle habits — can disrupt the digestive system and lead to pale stools. One common habit that affects Liver function is consistently staying awake between 11 pm and 3 am, the time when the Liver is most active according to the 24-hour wellness wheel. This is the period when the Liver works to store and cleanse the Blood, regulate Qi flow, and carry out detoxification and repair processes. If the body is not resting during this window, the Liver's ability to perform these tasks is diminished, which over time may weaken its capacity to produce and release bile — the substance responsible for giving stool its natural brown color. Beyond these functional imbalances, actual Liver diseases or infections like hepatitis or cirrhosis can directly impair bile production, leading to pale stools.

Damp-Heat obstructing the Gallbladder is another common TCM pattern linked to pale stools. In this condition, Dampness — a pathological accumulation of fluids — combines with Heat to create a thick, sticky obstruction within the Gallbladder and bile ducts. This blockage prevents bile from flowing freely into the intestines, causing stools to lose their normal color. In addition to pale stools, this pattern often presents with a bitter taste in the mouth, nausea, abdominal fullness or pain (especially on the right side), poor appetite, and sometimes jaundice (yellowing of the eyes or skin). Left unaddressed, Damp-Heat can harden into stones, further blocking bile flow and exacerbating digestive issues.

TCM also recognizes Blood Deficiency as a potential contributor to pale stools. Blood plays a vital nourishing role throughout your body, including your digestive system. A lack of adequate blood can indirectly influence stool color. Beyond internal imbalances, sometimes the cause simply can be external factors. Certain dietary choices, medications, supplements, or other substances you consume can temporarily affect stool color.

If you're noticing persistently pale stools, it's always a good idea to consult with a healthcare professional to understand the root cause and get the appropriate guidance.

Why Gallbladder And Liver Are Important To Our Body

You know, we often don't give much thought to our internal organs until something feels off. Yet, the Liver and Gallbladder are two incredibly vital and interconnected organs that profoundly influence both our physical health and emotional well-being.

Often seen as just a small pouch aiding digestion, the Gallbladder holds a deeper significance in TCM. Its most recognized physical role is to store and transport bile, a crucial digestive fluid produced by the Liver. Bile is essential for breaking down and absorbing fats and oils from your diet, ensuring you get the nutrients you need.

Beyond digestion, the Gallbladder is believed to be deeply connected to your mental and emotional state. In TCM, a well-functioning Gallbladder is linked to strong decision-making and sound judgment. It's also associated with the emotion of courage. If your Gallbladder energy is out of balance, you might find yourself struggling with fearfulness, timidity, or indecisiveness. Think of it as your inner compass and bravery barometer!

The Liver is a powerhouse organ, recognized in both TCM and Western medicine for its many responsibilities. In TCM, the Liver regulates Blood, Qi, and emotions. One of its key roles is storing and regulating Blood. Like a skilled logistics manager, it stores Blood at rest and dispatches it to the muscles, tissues, and organs during activity. This regulation supports smooth circulation and ensures the whole body receives proper nourishment.

The Liver is also intimately tied to your emotional well-being, particularly emotions like anger and frustration. When your Liver energy is unbalanced, it can manifest as mood swings, irritability, and general emotional instability. It's a key player in keeping your emotional landscape smooth and calm.

Furthermore, the Liver is the body's chief detoxification expert, processing and removing harmful toxins from your bloodstream. This role is universally acknowledged across medical traditions. Crucially, the Liver also governs the smooth flow of Qi throughout your entire body. If this flow is disrupted, you might experience a cascade of issues, from digestive problems and muscle tension to various aches and pains.

When the Liver and Gallbladder Are Out of Sync

When your Liver and Gallbladder aren't working in harmony, it can send ripples throughout your entire body, leading to a surprising array of symptoms. For starters, you might notice emotional disturbances. A disharmony between these two organs can significantly impact your mood, leading to irritability, mood swings, and a short temper. You might even experience feelings of depression, anxiety, or frustration.

Digestively, this imbalance can really throw things off. Since this system is vital for fat digestion, you might struggle with difficulty digesting fatty foods, indigestion, bloating, and discomfort after eating greasy meals. Other tell-tale signs can include belching, bloating, sour regurgitation, and changes in appetite.

The effects can even extend to your head and eyes. Liver disharmony often shows up as headaches, especially tension headaches. You might also notice various eye issues like blurry vision, redness, or dry eyes.

Physically, your muscles and joints can suffer. Because the Liver is responsible for the smooth flow of Qi, its disharmony can cause muscle tension, stiffness, and pain, particularly in your neck and shoulders. More broadly, this can lead to stagnation and blockage of Qi and Blood throughout your body, resulting in generalized pain, distension, and discomfort.

Sleep can also become elusive. An imbalanced Liver can contribute to various sleep disturbances, making it hard to fall asleep, causing you to wake up in the middle of the night, or leading to vivid dreams.

For women, this disharmony can impact menstrual and hormonal health. It might lead to irregular or painful periods, often aggravated by emotional stress. This imbalance can also disrupt overall hormonal balance, potentially contributing to conditions like premenstrual syndrome (PMS).

Even your skin can be a reflection of these internal imbalances, with conditions like acne or eczema sometimes linked to Liver issues in Traditional Chinese Medicine.

Understanding the profound importance of your organs and recognizing the signs of their imbalance are a crucial step towards maintaining holistic health and well-being. Have you noticed any of these symptoms in yourself?

Different Individuals May Experience Different Symptoms With Pale Or Clay-Colored Stool

Irritability. Individuals may experience mood swings, irritability, and emotional fluctuations. This is because the Liver is associated with the smooth flow of Qi in the body, and its dysfunction can result in emotional imbalances.

Digestive Issues. Liver and Gallbladder imbalances can lead to digestive problems, such as difficulty digesting fatty or greasy foods, resulting in discomfort after meals, bloating, belching, and flatulence.

Abdominal Discomfort. There may be discomfort or pain in the right upper abdomen where the Liver and Gallbladder are located. This pain can radiate to the back or shoulder and can be a red flag to seek medical assessment.

Frequent Bowel Movements. Often occurring soon after meals, indicating the Spleen's inability to transform and transport food efficiently.

Early-Morning Diarrhea. A hallmark symptom (sometimes called the "5 a.m. diarrhea") that may also occur during the night, caused by weakened Spleen Yang failing to warm and activate intestinal function.

Undigested Food Particles. A sign that food essence isn't being extracted properly, reflecting weak digestive fire and poor transformation.

Cold Sensation. During or after defecation, the individual may feel chilled, tired, or drained due to internal Cold and Qi depletion.

Pale, Bulky, or Watery Stool. Often lacking odor and occasionally containing mucus, this reflects Cold and Damp accumulation in the intestines.

Headaches. Individuals may experience headaches, especially on the sides of the head because the Gallbladder channel (energetic pathway) dominates the temporal and parietal regions of the head. These headaches are often described as a distending or throbbing sensation.

Eye Issues. Liver imbalances can affect the eyes, leading to symptoms like red, dry, or itchy eyes. Blurred vision or eye sensitivity to light may also occur.

Muscle Stiffness. As mentioned before, the Liver governs the tendons, so movement and flexibility may be impaired. Stiffness and tension in the neck and shoulders are most common.

Nausea and Vomiting. Some people may experience nausea or vomiting, particularly when gallstones are present.

Fatigue. People may feel tired, both physically and mentally.

Taste Changes. An unusual or bitter taste in the mouth may be experienced, which is often associated with Liver imbalances.

Yellowing of the Skin and Eyes (Jaundice). In more severe cases, Liver dysfunction can lead to jaundice, which is characterized by the yellowing of the skin and the whites of the eyes.

Sleep Disturbances. Difficulty staying asleep and needing or wanting to take a nap during the day are signs of Liver imbalance.

Self-Care and Support

Dietary Adjustments. Maintain a balanced and regular diet with a focus on fresh, whole foods. Include foods that nourish the Liver and Gallbladder, such as dark leafy greens, beets, artichokes, and bitter foods like dandelion greens. Reduce or avoid greasy, fried, spicy and processed foods, as well as excessive consumption of alcohol and caffeine.

Herbal Remedies. Consult with a TCM practitioner for herbal formulations tailored to your specific condition. Common herbs used to support Liver and Gallbladder health include milk thistle, dandelion, and turmeric.

Acupuncture. Acupuncture sessions can help restore the flow of Qi through the Liver and Gallbladder meridians. This can alleviate pain, improve mood, and promote overall well-being.

Qigong and Tai Chi. Engage in mind-body practices like Qigong and tai chi, which can help balance and harmonize the flow of Qi.

Stress Management. Explore stress-reduction techniques like meditation, deep breathing exercises, and mindfulness to manage emotional stress.

Lifestyle Modifications. Maintain a regular sleep schedule and prioritize quality sleep. Stay physically active through gentle exercises like walking or yoga. Address any unresolved emotional issues through therapy or counseling.

Massage. Massaging the lateral and medial sides of the leg, particularly mid-thigh and the area below the knee may help relieve tension and promote better energy flow.

Warm Compresses. Applying warm compresses to the right upper abdomen can help soothe the discomfort.

Regular Check-ups. If you suspect Gallbladder or Liver issues, consult with a TCM practitioner or a healthcare provider for a proper diagnosis and monitoring.

Foods To Relieve Gallbladder and Liver Dysfunction

Dark leafy greens. Vegetables like spinach, kale, and Swiss chard are rich in chlorophyll and can help cleanse the Liver. They also contain antioxidants that support Liver health.

Bitter greens. Bitter-tasting greens like dandelion greens, arugula, and mustard greens stimulate the Gallbladder and support bile production, aiding in digestion.

Beets. Beets are known for their Liver-cleansing properties. They contain betaine, which helps the Liver process fat, and pectin, which can help remove toxins.

Artichokes. Artichokes are excellent for Liver and Gallbladder health. They stimulate bile production, aiding in digestion and detoxification.

Turmeric. This spice contains curcumin, which has anti-inflammatory and antioxidant properties that benefit the Liver. It can help reduce inflammation and support overall Liver function.

Ginger. Ginger supports digestion and can reduce inflammation. It's beneficial for both the Liver and Gallbladder.

Milk thistle. While not a food, milk thistle is an herb known for its Liver-protective properties. Milk thistle brewed into an herbal tea is better than in supplement form.

Onions and garlic. These aromatic vegetables contain sulfur compounds that support Liver detoxification processes.

Lean protein. High-quality protein sources like chicken, turkey, and fish provide essential amino acids for Liver health.

Herbs. Herbs to support Liver and Gallbladder function, smooth Qi, and aid bile secretion include Curcuma Root (Yu Jin), Bupleurum Root (Chai Hu), Yin Chen Hao, and Gardenia Fruit (Zhi Zi). It is best to work with a qualified TCM practitioner when using herbal formulas. For daily support, herbal teas made from dandelion, or burdock root are known for their Liver-cleansing properties.

Whole grains. Choose whole grains like brown rice, quinoa, and oats, which provide sustained energy and fiber for healthy digestion.

Foods That Can Worsen Gallbladder and Liver Dysfunction

Fatty and fried foods. High-fat and deep-fried foods can overwhelm the Liver and Gallbladder, especially when dealing with dysfunction. Limit your intake of greasy foods like fast food, fried chicken, and fatty cuts of meat.

Processed foods. Processed foods often contain artificial additives, preservatives, and unhealthy trans fats that can strain the Liver and Gallbladder. This includes items like packaged snacks, sugary cereals, and convenience meals.

Excessive sugar. High sugar consumption can lead to a fatty Liver. Reduce your intake of sugary beverages, candies, pastries, and desserts.

Fruits. If you are experiencing pale stools, it is better to avoid fruit altogether until digestion improves, as raw and cooling foods can further weaken Spleen Yang and slow recovery.

Alcohol. Alcohol can put extra stress on the Liver. If you're dealing with dysfunction, it's best to limit or eliminate alcohol consumption.

Dairy products. Full-fat dairy products, particularly when consumed in excess, can contribute to Gallbladder problems and promote Dampness in the body. In TCM, dairy is considered cold and phlegm-producing, which can weaken the Spleen and impair digestion. If you are experiencing pale stools, it is best to avoid dairy entirely — even low-fat versions — until your digestion recovers. During this time, choose warm, easily digestible dairy alternatives such as oat milk or rice milk, served at room temperature or warmer.

Red meat. While lean protein sources are recommended, excessive consumption of red meat can burden the Liver and Gallbladder. Limit your intake and choose lean cuts.

Supplement and preservatives. Many supplements use starch, chemicals, or other binding agents with preservatives. Even vegetable capsules need chemicals to form the shape of the capsule. The chemicals and preservatives can cause more harm to the Liver.

Spicy foods. Very spicy foods can irritate the Gallbladder and Liver. If you're experiencing dysfunction, it's advisable to reduce spicy meals.

Soda and caffeinated beverages. Carbonated and caffeinated drinks may contribute to gallstone formation and place extra strain on digestion. Reducing or eliminating soda and coffee from your diet may help protect these organs. In particular, coffee can overstimulate already weakened Gallbladder and Liver function, leading to further imbalance.

Salty foods. In TCM, the salty flavor enters the Kidneys, and excessive salt intake can weaken Kidney Yin over time, indirectly affecting the Liver and Gallbladder. Too much salt can also contribute to fluid retention, thicken body fluids, and slow the free flow of Qi. Reduce your salt intake by avoiding heavily salted snacks and processed foods.

Sour foods. Sour foods in moderation, can help support the Liver — but excess sourness can overly constrain Qi, so balance is key.

Raw or cold foods. TCM advises against consuming raw or very cold foods, as they can weaken the digestive system, including the Liver and Gallbladder. Opt for warm, cooked meals.

16. Blood in The Stool With Or Without Pus And Mucus - Sign of bleeding in the lower portion of the digestive system with Intestinal Dampness and Heat

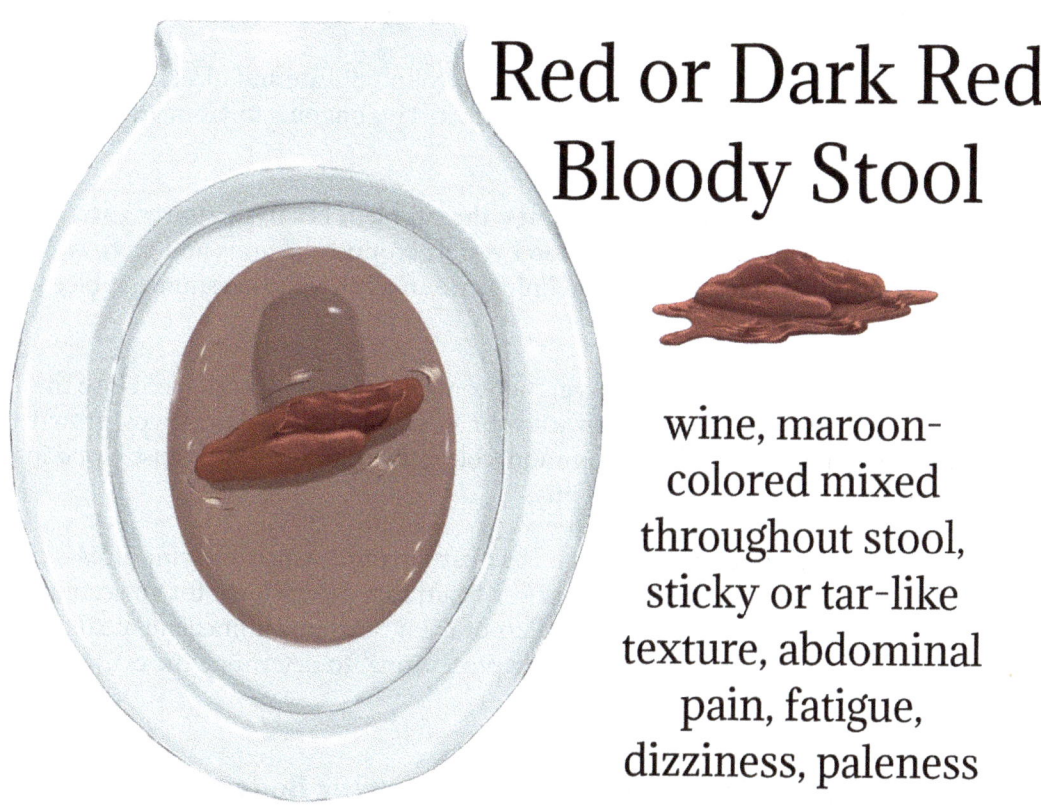

Red or Dark Red Bloody Stool

wine, maroon-colored mixed throughout stool, sticky or tar-like texture, abdominal pain, fatigue, dizziness, paleness

Figure 6.16 Red or dark red colored stool, Blood Heat, and Intestinal imbalance.

What it Means: In many cases, red stool is harmless and simply the result of eating naturally red foods — such as beets, red dragon fruit, or foods containing artificial red dyes — which temporarily change stool color without any actual bleeding. However, when bright red blood appears on, around or mixed in the stool, especially if it is visible on toilet paper or in the toilet water, it may indicate bleeding in the lower part of the digestive tract. This fresh blood is most often associated with the rectum, anus, or lower colon. Darker red stool, on the other hand, may suggest bleeding slightly higher in the large intestine. In Traditional Chinese Medicine, such bleeding is often linked to Heat in the Blood, Damp-Heat in the Large Intestine, or Qi not holding the Blood properly, all of which can irritate or damage intestinal blood vessels.

Underlying Causes

Seeing blood, mucus, or pus in your stool can be alarming, and in Traditional Chinese Medicine, this often points to an Intestinal Damp-Heat pattern — a specific internal imbalance with multiple possible triggers, ranging from dietary habits to chronic health conditions. In this pattern, the intestines become a warm, humid environment where fluids thicken and stagnate. This combination of Dampness and Heat irritates the intestinal lining, disrupting the smooth flow of Qi and causing inflammation. As a result, stool color and consistency change, and blood, mucus, or pus may appear. This internal imbalance is often aggravated by poor eating habits, such as frequent consumption of greasy or spicy foods, irregular meal times, or overeating. In TCM theory, spicy foods tend to create Heat, while rich, oily foods generate Dampness — together forming the Damp-Heat pattern that inflames and injures the intestinal walls.

While diet plays a significant role, other factors can ignite or contribute to this Intestinal Damp-Heat pattern:

- Infections or Inflammatory Conditions: Any infection or inflammatory condition affecting your gastrointestinal system can wreak havoc, irritating and damaging the intestinal lining. This direct damage is a common reason for blood, mucus, and pus appearing in your stool.

- Intestinal Parasitic Infections: Tiny invaders like certain intestinal parasites can directly harm your intestinal lining, causing bleeding and often leading to mucus in your stool.

- Inflammatory Bowel Disease (IBD): Conditions like Crohn's disease and ulcerative colitis, both forms of IBD, involve chronic inflammation of the digestive tract. This ongoing inflammation is a significant cause of blood, mucus, and pus in the stool.

- Structural Issues in the Lower Tract: Sometimes, the problem lies in the lower parts of your digestive system. Hemorrhoids, which are swollen blood vessels around the anus and rectum, can bleed when irritated. Anal fissures, small tears in the anal lining, are another common source of bleeding, sometimes with mucus.

- Ulcers and Growths: Gastrointestinal ulcers in the Stomach or Intestines can bleed into the digestive tract, potentially mixing blood, mucus, and pus with your stool. Similarly, colon polyps, growths on the inner lining of the colon, can bleed. While less common, colorectal cancer can also cause blood in the stool and, in advanced stages, may involve mucus and pus.

Understanding these diverse causes of Intestinal Damp Heat patterns and associated symptoms is crucial. If you're experiencing any of these signs, it's always best to consult a healthcare professional for an accurate diagnosis and appropriate treatment. Any blood in your stool, regardless of color, warrants immediate medical attention. It's a symptom that should always be evaluated by a healthcare professional to determine the cause and ensure proper treatment.

How Dampness And Heat In The Intestines Can Affect Our Body

When your body experiences what Traditional Chinese Medicine calls Intestinal Damp-Heat, it's like a swampy, overheated condition brewing within your digestive system. This internal imbalance can trigger a cascade of uncomfortable symptoms, affecting not just your gut but your overall well-being.

The most direct impact of Intestinal Damp-Heat is on digestion. You may experience persistent diarrhea or loose stools, often accompanied by abdominal discomfort, bloating, and a heavy sensation in the abdomen. The stools themselves can be revealing — they may appear greasy, sticky, or have a distinctly foul odor. This combination of internal Heat and Dampness can also cause frequent urges to defecate, often leaving you with the uncomfortable sensation of not having fully emptied your bowels. While diarrhea is common in this pattern, it can also cause irregular bowel habits, leading to frustrating cycles of alternating diarrhea and constipation.

The influence of Intestinal Damp-Heat doesn't stop at your digestive tract. The internal heat can manifest as excessive thirst and a dry mouth, as your body tries to signal its need for fluids to cool down. This imbalance can also show up on your skin, leading to issues like acne, rashes, or redness, as TCM often links skin problems to internal disharmonies.

You might find yourself feeling surprisingly fatigued and lethargic. That's because your body's energy is constantly diverted to combat this internal imbalance, leaving you feeling drained. The heat can also impact your urinary system, causing burning during urination or an increased frequency of urination. Even your mood can be affected, with individuals often experiencing irritability or mood swings due to the ongoing discomfort and disrupted internal harmony.

A TCM practitioner would likely confirm this pattern by observing a thick, yellow coating on your tongue, a classic diagnostic sign reflecting the presence of Damp-Heat within your system. Recognizing these varied symptoms can be the first step toward addressing red, bloody stool and restoring balance to your body.

Different Individuals May Experience Different Symptoms With Blood in The Stool With Or Without Pus And Mucus

Bright Red Blood. Bright red blood in the stool often suggests bleeding in the lower digestive tract, such as the rectum or the colon. This can result from conditions like hemorrhoids, anal fissures, or diverticulosis.

Bloody Diarrhea. If you experience diarrhea with blood in the stool, it may be linked to inflammatory bowel diseases (IBD) like Crohn's disease or ulcerative colitis, infections, or other gastrointestinal conditions.

Presence of Mucus. The presence of mucus in the stool is often seen in conditions like irritable bowel syndrome (IBS) or infections. Mucus can sometimes accompany blood in the stool.

Abdominal Pain. Abdominal pain, cramping, or discomfort is a common symptom that can accompany blood in the stool. The location and severity of the pain may provide clues about the underlying cause.

Change in Bowel Habits. Blood in the stool may be associated with changes in bowel habits, such as diarrhea, constipation, or alternating episodes of both.

Fatigue. Chronic blood loss through the stool can lead to anemia, resulting in fatigue, weakness, and pallor.

Weight Loss. Unexplained weight loss may occur in some cases, especially if the underlying condition affects nutrient absorption or metabolism.

Fever. Fever may be accompanied by other whole-body signs of illness, indicating that the cause of blood in the stool might be more serious or widespread.

Painful Bowel Movements. Conditions like anal fissures or hemorrhoids may cause pain and discomfort during bowel movements.

Self Care and Support

Consult a Healthcare Professional. The first and most crucial step is to consult a healthcare professional, such as a gastroenterologist, to determine the underlying cause of the symptoms. They will conduct necessary tests, examinations, and assessments to identify the specific condition and recommend appropriate treatment.

Stay Hydrated. If you experience diarrhea along with blood in the stool, it's essential to stay well-hydrated. Dehydration can result from fluid loss due to diarrhea, and adequate hydration is important for your overall health.

Maintain a Food Diary. Keeping a food diary can help you and your healthcare provider identify potential triggers or food sensitivities that may be contributing to your symptoms. Note the foods you consume and any changes in symptoms you observe.

Modify Diet. Your healthcare provider may recommend specific dietary changes or restrictions based on your diagnosis. In some cases, a diet low in certain types of fiber, spicy foods, or other dietary triggers may be advised.

Consume More Fiber. For certain conditions like hemorrhoids or diverticulosis, increased dietary fiber or fiber supplements may be recommended to promote regular bowel movements and reduce the risk of further irritation.

Take Prescribed Medications. Depending on the diagnosis, your healthcare provider may prescribe medications such as antibiotics for infections, anti-inflammatory drugs for inflammatory conditions, or other medications to manage specific symptoms.

Address Stress. High levels of stress can exacerbate gastrointestinal symptoms. Consider stress-reduction techniques like relaxation exercises, meditation, or yoga.

Follow-Up with Physician. Attend regular follow-up appointments with your healthcare provider to monitor your progress and adjust your treatment plan as needed.

Avoid Self-Diagnosis and Self-Treatment. It's important not to attempt self-diagnosis or self-treatment for these symptoms. While certain over-the-counter medications can help alleviate minor discomfort, they should not be used as a substitute for professional medical advice.

Learn More and Seek Support. Seek information and support from reliable sources or patient advocacy organizations related to your specific condition. Understanding your diagnosis and having a support system can be beneficial during your healthcare journey.

Foods To Relieve Dampness And Heat In The Intestines

Cooling foods. Water-rich fruits and vegetables like cucumbers, watermelon, and leafy greens counteract heat in the body.

Herbs. Herbs to clear Damp-Heat, cool Blood, and stop bleeding include Platycladus orientalis (Ce Bai Ye), Scute (Huang Qin), Angelica Tails (Dang Gui Wei), and Fructus Sophorae (Huai Hua). It is best to work with a qualified TCM practitioner when using herbal formulas. For daily support, herbal teas such as chrysanthemum tea or mint tea. These can have a cooling and soothing effect on the digestive system.

Whole grains. Choose whole grains like brown rice, quinoa, and oats. These are less likely to create dampness in the intestines compared to refined grains.

Lean proteins. Opt for lean protein sources like skinless poultry, fish, and tofu. Avoid fatty cuts of meat.

Digestive-friendly herbs. Incorporate herbs like lotus roots and pear into your cooking. They can aid digestion and have a mild cooling effect.

Plenty of water. Stay well-hydrated by drinking plain room temperature water. Proper hydration helps maintain a healthy balance in the intestines.

Steamed and lightly cooked foods. Opt for cooking methods like steaming, stir-frying, or lightly boiling your vegetables and foods. These methods are less likely to create excess Dampness and Heat compared to deep frying or grilling.

Foods That Can Worsen Dampness And Heat In The Intestinal

Spicy foods. Hot peppers, chili, and other spicy foods can increase Heat in the Intestines.

Greasy and fried foods. Fried foods, fast food, and heavily greasy items can exacerbate Dampness and Heat.

Processed sugars. Excessive consumption of sugary foods, including candies, pastries, and sweet beverages, can contribute to Dampness.

Dairy. Dairy products, especially full-fat varieties, can create Dampness in the body for some individuals. While low-fat or lactose-free options may be tolerated better, they can still be difficult for the Spleen to process. In general, even people with otherwise healthy digestion may find that regular dairy consumption gradually weakens their system over time.

Refined grains. Refined grains like white rice, white bread, and pasta can worsen Dampness. Opt for whole grains instead.

Alcohol. Alcohol can generate Heat and Dampness in the body. Limit your alcohol intake.

Caffeine. Caffeinated beverages, such as coffee and certain teas, are both drying and heat-producing in nature. From a TCM perspective, they can deplete Yin and fluids, while overstimulating Yang. For this reason, it's best to limit or avoid caffeine consumption, especially if you already struggle with dryness, heat, or weak digestion.

Excessive cold foods. While cooling foods can help, consuming too many very cold or raw foods can potentially damage the Spleen and create Dampness. Moderation is key.

Heavy meats. Fatty and red meats can contribute to Heat and Dampness. Choose lean protein sources.

Excessive salt. High-salt foods can promote dampness. Watch your sodium intake.

Moldy or spoiled foods. Foods that have gone bad, or moldy items, can generate Dampness and Heat when consumed.

Overeating. Consuming large quantities of food in one sitting can overwhelm the digestive system and create Dampness. Eat in moderation.

Processed and preserved foods. Processed foods, canned goods, and items with artificial additives may contribute to Dampness and Heat.

Excessive sweets. Overloading on sweets, even fruit juices, can lead to Dampness. Stick to reasonable portions of naturally sweet foods.

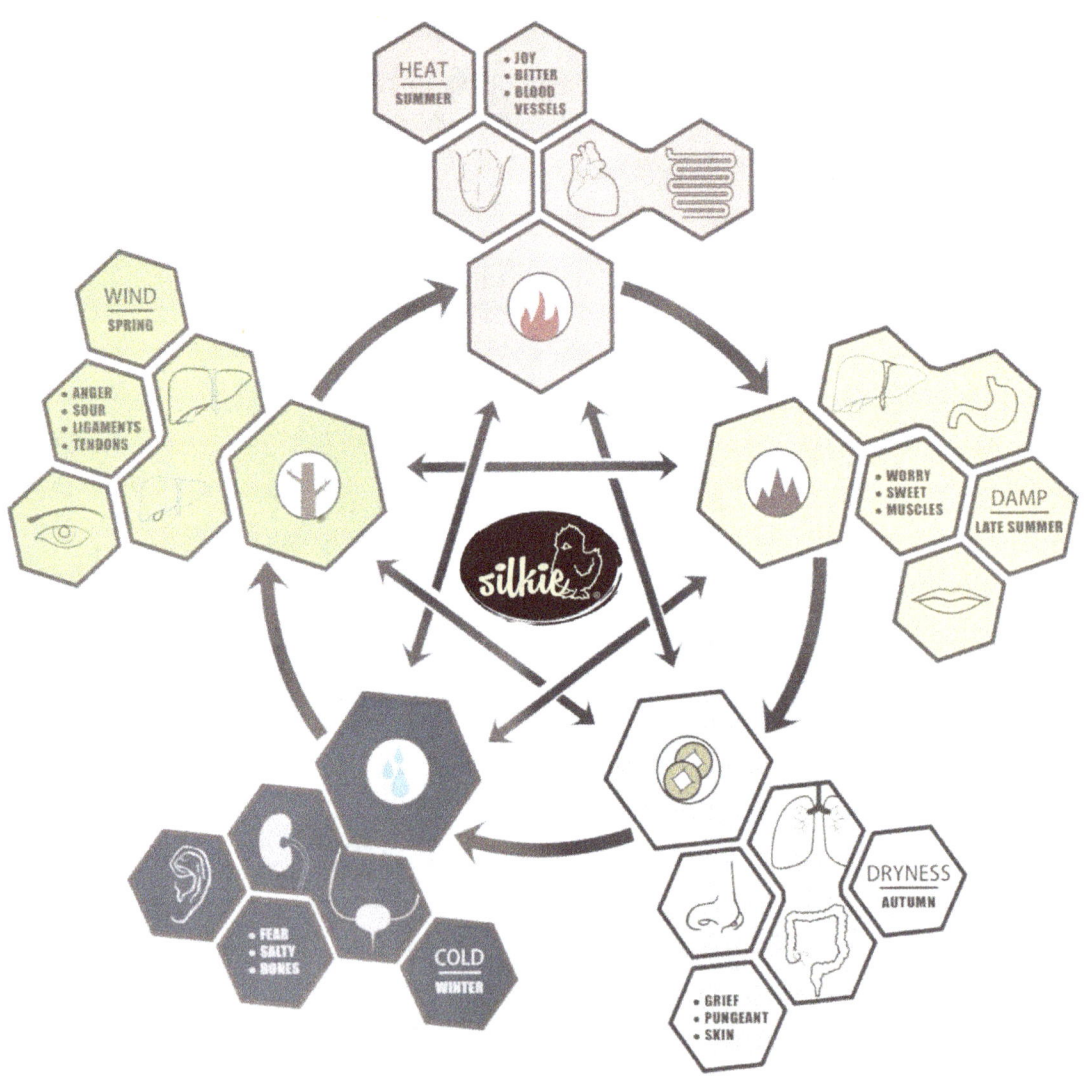

17. Black Tar-Like Or Dark Purple Bloody Stool - Sign of bleeding in the upper digestive tract with deficiency of the Spleen and Stomach

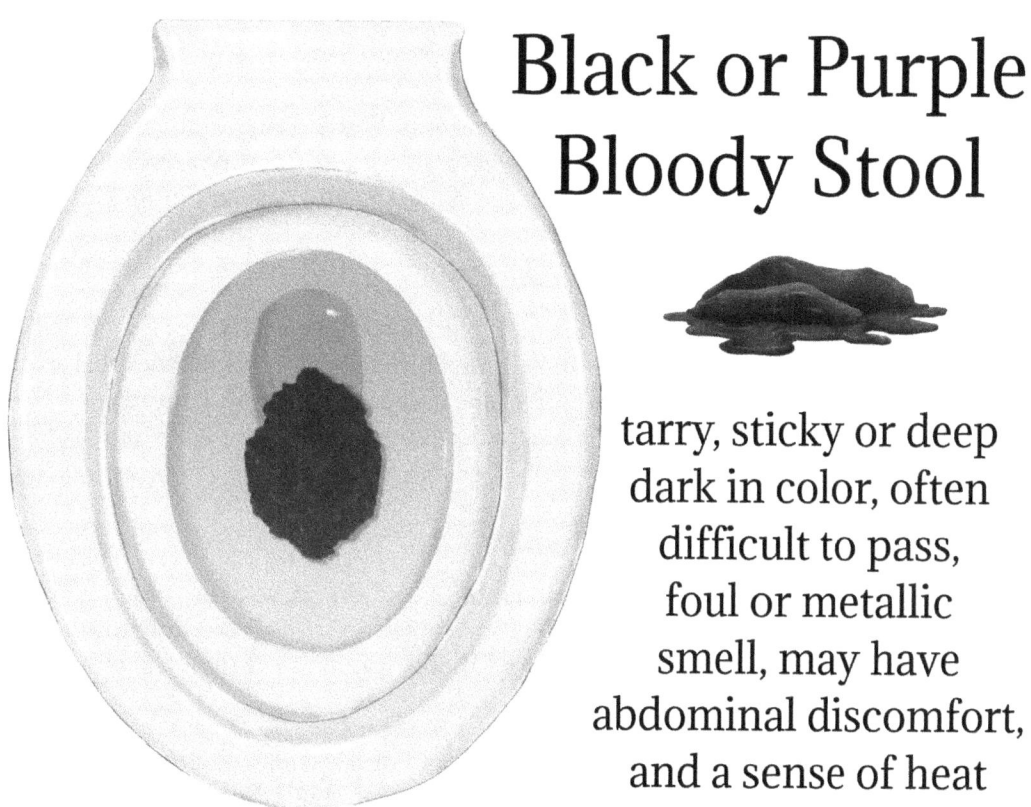

Figure 6.17 Black colored stool, Spleen Qi Deficiency, Liver Qi Stagnation, Blood Stasis, or chronic Heat in the Stomach or Intestines.

What it Means: When stool appears black, tarry, or unusually dark, it is almost always a sign of bleeding somewhere in the upper digestive tract (stomach, esophagus, or small intestine). From a Western view, this is called melena and often results from ulcers, gastritis, varices, or medication effects (like NSAIDs). The black color appears because blood has been partially digested before exiting.

In Traditional Chinese Medicine (TCM), black stool may arise from two broad categories of imbalance: Deficiency patterns and Excess patterns.

Deficiency-type black stool: Often linked to Spleen and Stomach Qi (or Yang) Deficiency, where weak digestive Qi fails to hold Blood within the vessels. This slow leakage, combined with weak transformation, allows blood to seep into the stool. People with this pattern often appear pale, fatigued, cold in the hands and feet, with poor appetite, bloating, and palpitations. In this case, the black stool reflects a system too weak to contain Blood properly.

Excess-type black stool: More acute and forceful, usually tied to Liver Qi Stagnation, Blood Stasis, or Chronic Heat in the Stomach/Intestines.

Liver Qi Stagnation builds pressure, constraining the digestive tract and disrupting Blood circulation. Over time, this stress may force Blood out of the vessels.

Blood Stasis makes Blood thick, dark, and sluggish, weakening vessel walls and creating clotted, tar-like stools.

Chronic Heat agitates Blood and causes it to move recklessly, damaging vessel linings and leading to bleeding that darkens as it passes through the gut.

Together, these patterns explain why black stool in TCM is never viewed in isolation. It can mean weakness (a system unable to hold Blood) or excess (Heat and stagnation forcing Blood out).

Underlying Causes

Upper gastrointestinal (GI) bleeding is always a serious concern. In Western medicine, the most common causes include peptic ulcers in the stomach or duodenum, severe gastritis, and gastroesophageal reflux disease (GERD). Medications such as non-steroidal anti-inflammatory drugs (NSAIDs) and corticosteroids can irritate and erode the stomach lining, while chronic Helicobacter pylori infection is a frequent culprit for ulcer formation. Systemic clotting disorders, such as hemophilia, also make upper GI bleeding more likely.

From a Traditional Chinese Medicine perspective, however, black or tar-like stool is not simply about the physical bleeding itself but about the pattern of imbalance that allowed bleeding to occur. Rather than treating only the ulcer or inflamed tissue, TCM aims to identify and correct the deeper disharmony. Four major TCM patterns are most often involved: Spleen Qi Deficiency, Liver Qi Stagnation, Blood Stasis, and Chronic Heat in the Stomach or Intestines.

Spleen Qi Deficiency

In TCM, the Spleen is responsible for transforming food into Qi and Blood, and for "holding" Blood within the vessels. When Spleen Qi is weak, this containment function is impaired, making bleeding more likely. Over time, the weakened Spleen struggles to produce sufficient Qi and Blood, leading to chronic deficiency and a body that tires easily.

Symptoms of this pattern often include fatigue, poor appetite, abdominal distention after meals, loose or unformed stools, and a pale complexion. Patients may also have cold hands and feet, sluggishness, and easy bruising not caused by medications. In the case of black stool, bleeding occurs because the vessels are no longer firmly supported by the Spleen's Qi, allowing blood to leak into the digestive tract.

This pattern frequently overlaps with Western findings such as anemia, peptic ulcers, or chronic gastritis. But while Western treatment may focus on stopping the bleeding itself, TCM emphasizes strengthening the Spleen so the problem does not return.

Liver Qi Stagnation

The Liver's role in TCM is to ensure the smooth flow of Qi and Blood throughout the body. When emotional stress, frustration, or repressed anger accumulates, the Liver's Qi becomes constrained. This stagnation disrupts circulation, creating pressure in the digestive tract and making its vessels more vulnerable to rupture.

Symptoms often include digestive discomfort that worsens under stress, a sense of distention or pain under the ribs, irritability, mood swings, and irregular bowel movements. If bleeding occurs, it may present as dark or tarry stool, sometimes alongside abdominal cramping.

In Western medicine, this is often seen in stress-related ulcers, irritable bowel syndrome with bleeding, or flare-ups of chronic inflammatory conditions. Treatment in TCM focuses on soothing the Liver, regulating emotions, and restoring the free flow of Qi so that pressure is relieved and bleeding does not recur.

Blood Stasis

When circulation remains blocked for a long time, stagnation of Qi can harden into Blood Stasis. This means Blood becomes thick, dark, and sluggish, much like traffic coming to a standstill on a crowded road. The result is pressure and congestion in the digestive tract, where fragile vessels may rupture and cause chronic or recurrent bleeding.

Symptoms of Blood Stasis include sharp or stabbing abdominal pain, fixed areas of discomfort, dark or purplish lips or complexion, and a tongue that appears dark with purple spots. The stool itself may appear very dark, sticky, and tar-like, reflecting the congealed nature of the bleeding.

Western diagnoses may include chronic ulcers that do not heal, scarring or narrowing in the digestive tract, or complications from long-term liver disease. TCM treatment emphasizes invigorating the Blood, dispersing stasis, and improving circulation so that pressure on vessels is relieved and new bleeding is prevented.

Chronic Heat in the Stomach or Intestines

If weakness and stagnation are not the root, Heat damaging the digestive tract is another common cause of black stool. This Heat can arise from internal imbalances such as Stomach Yin Deficiency (a lack of cooling, nourishing fluids), or from lifestyle habits like frequent alcohol consumption, heavy use of spicy or greasy foods, or chronic stress that fuels internal fire.

Over time, this Heat irritates the mucosal lining of the stomach and intestines, inflames the tissues, and damages the blood vessels, leading to bleeding that appears as black or tarry stool. Symptoms include burning or gnawing abdominal pain, thirst, bad breath, irritability, a red tongue with yellow coating, and a strong preference for cold drinks.

In Western medicine, this correlates with chronic gastritis, acid reflux, and peptic ulcers aggravated by diet and lifestyle. Treatment in TCM involves clearing Heat, nourishing Yin, and protecting the stomach lining to reduce further damage.

Black stool is always a warning sign that requires medical attention. In Western medicine, it demands urgent investigation to rule out ulcers, gastrointestinal bleeding, or cancer. In TCM, it is equally seen as a marker of deep systemic imbalance — whether from weakness of the Spleen, stagnation of the Liver, congealed Blood, or Heat damaging the digestive tract.

A skilled TCM practitioner looks at the entire constellation of symptoms: fatigue and bruising point toward Spleen Qi Deficiency; irritability and rib pain suggest Liver Qi Stagnation; stabbing abdominal pain with sticky black stool signals Blood Stasis; while burning pain and thirst reflect chronic Stomach or Intestinal Heat. Treatment is tailored to the root cause, using herbal formulas to stop bleeding, acupuncture to move Qi and Blood, and dietary adjustments to rebuild digestive strength.

By addressing both the immediate bleeding and the underlying imbalance, TCM not only seeks to resolve black stool but also to restore long-term harmony, preventing recurrence and strengthening the body from within.

How Bleeding in the Upper Digestive Tract Can Affect Our Body

When bleeding begins in the upper digestive tract, the immediate concern is blood loss — but in TCM, the effects go far deeper, reflecting how the core organ systems are weakened and thrown out of balance.

Qi and Blood are inseparable: Qi generates Blood, while Blood serves as the carrier for Qi. When bleeding occurs, both are depleted at once. This loss undermines vitality and weakens the body's ability to function, leaving patients fatigued, pale, dizzy, and unable to concentrate. Because Qi is diminished, warmth and energy production falter, leading to chills, cold extremities, and slowed recovery after illness.

The Spleen, which governs the production of Blood and ensures that it stays within the vessels, is hit especially hard. Each episode of bleeding not only drains Blood but also further weakens the Spleen's transformative power. As digestion slows, appetite decreases, stools may turn loose or unformed, and fatigue worsens. A vicious cycle sets in: the weaker the Spleen, the less it can hold Blood, and the more bleeding occurs.

The Liver is also implicated, especially when bleeding is linked to emotional strain. Stagnant Liver Qi disrupts the free flow of energy and drains the Liver's Blood stores. Without sufficient Blood to anchor the Shen (spirit), patients often experience irritability, headaches, restless sleep, or emotional instability. Women may also see changes in menstruation.

If bleeding becomes chronic, Blood Stasis inevitably develops. Sluggish circulation thickens and congeals Blood, creating sharp or stabbing abdominal pain and leaving tissues undernourished. Extremities may feel cold or heavy, ulcers heal slowly, and patients are left with long-lasting fatigue and stiffness.

When Heat is the driver, as in cases of Stomach or Intestinal Heat, the problem is compounded. Heat agitates the Blood, damages vessel linings, and dries up Yin fluids, worsening both bleeding and systemic weakness. Patients may complain of burning abdominal pain, foul breath, thirst, or irritability, with a red tongue and yellow coating. Over time, persistent Heat not only irritates but also accelerates aging by depleting the body's deeper reserves.

Ultimately, upper digestive bleeding is never just a local issue. Whether rooted in Spleen weakness, Liver stagnation, Blood Stasis, or Heat, the systemic consequences are clear: lowered vitality, compromised digestion, emotional instability, weakened circulation, and reduced immunity. For this reason, TCM treatment emphasizes more than stopping bleeding. It focuses on restoring harmony, strengthening the organs, nourishing Qi and Blood, and clearing pathogenic factors to prevent recurrence — a holistic approach that seeks not only immediate relief but also long-term resilience.

Different Individuals May Experience Different Symptoms With Dark Purple or Black Tar-Like Color Bloody Stool

Black Tar-Like Stool. This stool color is often associated with the presence of old blood in the digestive tract. It may suggest bleeding from the upper digestive system, including the stomach or the upper part of the small intestine.

Excessive Heat or Heat in the Blood. TCM considers this stool color as a sign of excessive heat in the digestive system or Heat in the Blood. Excessive heat can result from consuming hot and spicy foods, and emotional stress. This is a pattern of heat in the body.

Digestive Discomfort. Symptoms associated with this stool color may manifest as abdominal pain, a feeling of fullness or discomfort in the stomach, acid regurgitation, and a bitter taste in the mouth.

Poor Appetite. The presence of black, tar-like stool may be accompanied by a loss of appetite due to discomfort in the digestive system.

Foul Odor. The stool often has a distinct and unusually foul smell due to the presence of old blood.

Abdominal Pain. Pain or discomfort in the abdomen is common, especially if there is bleeding from ulcers or inflammation in the stomach or intestines.

Fatigue or Weakness. Blood loss over time can lead to anemia, causing fatigue, weakness, or dizziness.

Nausea and Vomiting. Some people may experience nausea or vomiting, especially if there's a significant issue in the stomach or intestines.

Pale or Cold Skin. Due to blood loss, skin may appear pale, or there may be coldness in extremities.

Shortness of Breath. Severe or prolonged blood loss may result in shortness of breath or a rapid heart rate.

Self-Care and Support

Seek Medical Attention. If you notice black, tarry stools, or any unusual stool color, it's essential to consult a healthcare professional or a gastroenterologist promptly. This is especially critical if you experience other symptoms, such as abdominal pain or fatigue.

Follow Medical Advice. Once diagnosed, it's important to follow the treatment plan recommended by your healthcare provider. Treatment will depend on the underlying cause, which may involve addressing issues like gastrointestinal bleeding, stomach ulcers, or other digestive problems.

Modify Diet. Avoid foods and beverages that can irritate the stomach or digestive tract, such as spicy, acidic, or greasy foods.

Take Medicine. If prescribed medication, make sure to take it as directed by your healthcare provider. Medications for stomach ulcers, gastrointestinal bleeding, or other related issues will play a significant role in your recovery.

Stay Hydrated. It's important to stay well-hydrated, especially if you experience bleeding. Ensure you drink enough fluids to maintain your body's fluid balance.

Rest and Recover. If you're experiencing fatigue or anemia due to blood loss, ensure you get adequate rest to support your body's healing process.

Monitor Symptoms. Keep track of any changes in your symptoms or stool color, and report them to your healthcare provider. Regular follow-up appointments may be necessary to assess your progress.

Find Emotional Support. Coping with health concerns can be emotionally challenging. Seek support from friends, family, or a counselor to help manage stress and anxiety.

Foods To Relieve Bleeding In The Upper Digestive Tract

Easy-to-digest grains. Opt for easily digestible grains such as rice, congee (rice porridge), and oats. These grains are gentle on the digestive system and can provide nourishment without overtaxing the Spleen and Stomach.

Cooked vegetables. Cooked and steamed vegetables are easier to digest than raw ones. Choose mild, non-gassy options like carrots, zucchini, and green beans.

Lean protein. Lean sources of protein, such as skinless poultry, white fish, and tofu, are less likely to irritate the digestive tract. They can provide essential nutrients without adding extra strain.

Fruits. Opt for well-cooked or ripe fruits that are easy to digest, such as apples, pears, and bananas. Avoid very acidic or citrus fruits that may be harsh on the stomach.

Herbs. Herbs to strengthen the Spleen, stop bleeding, and cool Blood include Codonopsis (Dang Shen), Angelica Root (Dang Gui), Notoginseng root (Tianqi), and Lotus Rhizome Node (Ou Jie). It is best to work with a qualified TCM practitioner when using herbal formulas. For daily support, herbal teas such as ginger can help soothe the digestive system related to cold and chamomile teas can help soothe the digestive system related to heat. A small amount of turmeric, in particular, is known for its ability to reduce inflammation and support digestion.

Mild spices. Use gentle warming spices such as fennel, cumin, and coriander. In TCM, these spices help support the Spleen and Stomach, improving digestion without creating excess Heat or Dampness. They add flavor to green vegetables and meals while being kind to the digestive system.

Bone broth. Bone broth is gentle on the stomach and provides essential nutrients that support overall health.

Room temperature water. Drink plenty of water to stay well-hydrated, especially if there's bleeding involved.

Foods That Can Worsen Bleeding In The Upper Digestive Tract

Spicy foods. Spicy foods, including hot peppers and strong spices, can further irritate the digestive tract and contribute to bleeding.

Greasy and fried foods. These can be difficult to digest and may lead to more discomfort and bleeding in the upper digestive tract.

Citrus and acidic foods. Citrus fruits and highly acidic foods like tomatoes and vinegar can be harsh on the stomach lining, potentially worsening symptoms.

Alcohol. Alcohol can aggravate the stomach lining, leading to more irritation and potentially make bleeding worse.

Caffeine. Caffeinated beverages like coffee and certain teas can stimulate acid production in the stomach, which may exacerbate bleeding.

Processed and spicy condiments. Condiments like ketchup, hot sauces, and processed marinades are often high in spices and additives that can irritate the stomach.

Dairy products. Some individuals with Spleen and Stomach Deficiency may have difficulty digesting lactose. In general, even people with otherwise healthy digestion may find that regular dairy consumption could lead to gastrointestinal discomfort and gradually weakens their system over time.

Large meals. Overeating or consuming large meals can place additional stress on the digestive system. Opt for smaller, more frequent meals.

Hard-to-digest foods. Tough meats, raw vegetables, and foods high in fiber may be hard to digest, potentially worsening the condition.

Artificial additives. Artificial colors, flavors, and preservatives found in many processed foods can contribute to stomach discomfort.

Excessively cold or icy foods. Very cold or icy foods and beverages can shock the digestive system and should be consumed in moderation.

Sugary foods and sodas. Excessive sugar intake can potentially disrupt digestive processes. It's best to limit sugary foods and drinks.

Large amounts of red meat. Large quantities of red meat can be hard to digest and may lead to stomach discomfort.

Unripe or extremely sour fruits. Unripe or extremely sour fruits can be harsh on the stomach lining.

18. Bright Red Blood - Sign of severe Liver disease or variceal bleeding

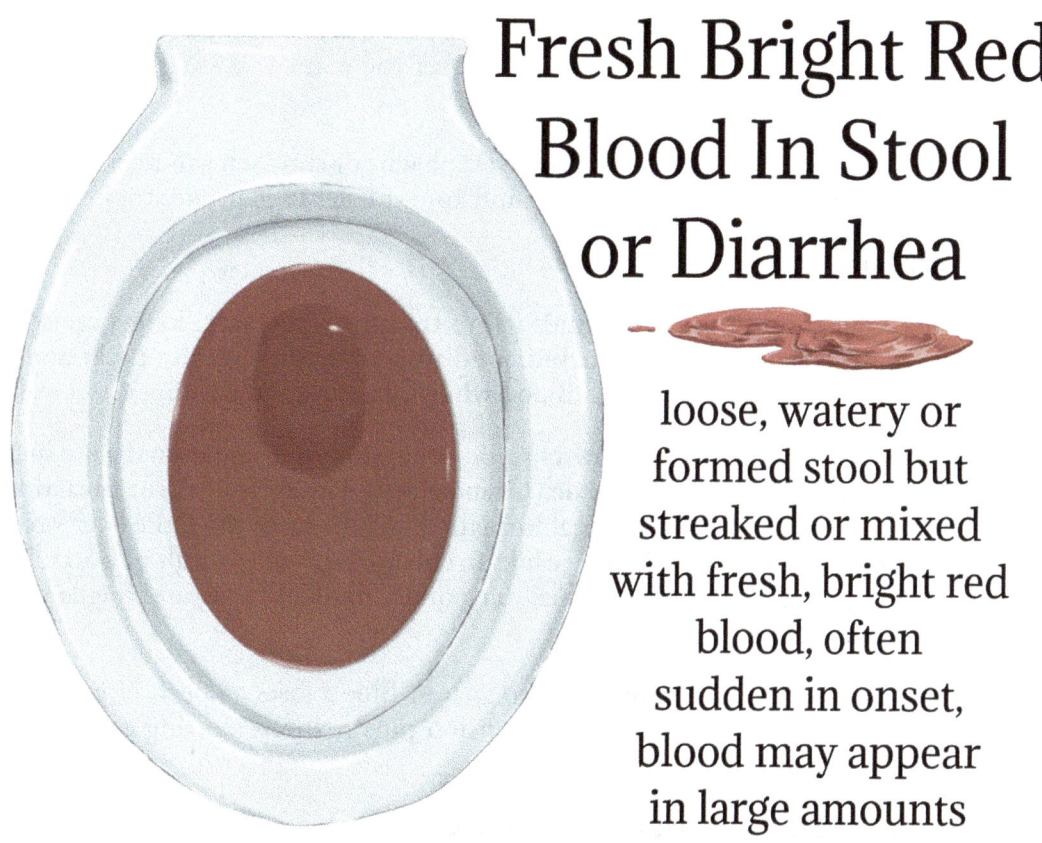

Fresh Bright Red Blood In Stool or Diarrhea — loose, watery or formed stool but streaked or mixed with fresh, bright red blood, often sudden in onset, blood may appear in large amounts

Figure 6.18 Fresh bright red blood in stool or diarrhea, chronic Liver Qi Stagnation, Damp-Heat accumulation, and Blood Stasis damaging the Liver collaterals, gradually leading to vessel fragility and bleeding.

What it Means: When bright red blood appears in the stool — not just as streaks but in larger amounts, sometimes mixed with diarrhea — it may indicate severe bleeding from the digestive tract due to advanced liver disease, such as cirrhosis. In cirrhosis, scarring of the liver can obstruct blood flow, leading to dangerously enlarged veins (varices) in the esophagus or stomach. If these varices rupture, they can cause sudden, heavy bleeding that may pass through the digestive tract and appear as bright red blood in the stool. This is a medical emergency and requires immediate hospital care.

From a Traditional Chinese Medicine perspective, cirrhosis and variceal bleeding are often linked to long-term stagnation of Liver Qi and Blood, transforming into Heat and Dryness, which damages the Blood vessels. Over time, this chronic disharmony weakens the Liver's ability to store blood and maintain smooth circulation, leading to sudden leakage of blood outside its normal pathways.

Underlying Causes

Advanced Liver Disease: Cirrhosis caused by chronic hepatitis, alcohol-related liver damage, or non-alcoholic fatty liver disease can increase pressure in the portal vein system (portal hypertension), leading to the formation of fragile varices that can rupture. Once varices form, even minor increases in pressure — such as from coughing, vomiting, or straining during bowel movements — can cause them to bleed. This bleeding may appear as bright red blood in the stool or black, tarry stools if the bleeding is higher up in the digestive tract. Left untreated, variceal bleeding can become life-threatening and often requires urgent medical care.

First TCM Factor: Chronic Liver Qi Stagnation

In TCM, the Liver is responsible for ensuring the smooth flow of Qi throughout the body. When Qi movement in the Liver becomes blocked over time — due to emotional stress, poor diet, or long-term illness — the stagnation creates internal tension and pressure. This pressure not only affects emotional health but also disrupts Blood flow in the Liver and nearby vessels. Over the years, this stuck Qi can transform into Heat, damaging tissues and blood vessels.

Variceal Rupture: The bursting of enlarged veins in the esophagus or stomach can release large amounts of blood into the digestive tract, which may pass quickly and appear bright red in the stool.

Second TCM Factor: Damp-Heat Accumulation

When the Liver cannot maintain smooth flow, fluids fail to transform properly. Excess moisture combines with Heat, creating Damp-Heat — a sticky, turbid condition that congests the Liver and Gallbladder channels. In TCM, this stagnation blocks Qi and Blood while inflaming and eroding vessel walls.

From a biomedical perspective, this mirrors how chronic congestion and inflammation damage both endothelial linings (blood vessel walls) and liver tissue (parenchyma). The cycle of tissue breakdown and scarring (fibrosis) raises portal pressure, fueling variceal formation. At the same time, the liver's reduced ability to produce clotting proteins weakens coagulation, while an enlarged spleen (a result of portal hypertension) traps platelets, worsening clotting failure. The result: veins under immense pressure, fragile walls, and poor clotting — a perfect storm for catastrophic bleeding.

In TCM terms, Damp-Heat clogs the channels, Qi stagnates, Blood loses smooth circulation, and vessel integrity weakens. In biomedical terms, portal hypertension plus reduced clotting capacity explains why variceal bleeding is both sudden and difficult to control.

Third TCM Factor: Blood Stasis Damaging the Liver Collaterals

In TCM, "collaterals" refer to the network of smaller vessels and channels that distribute Blood throughout the body. Long-term Qi stagnation and Damp-Heat eventually slow the Blood so much that it becomes stagnant — a condition called "Blood Stasis." Stagnant Blood puts constant strain on the vessel walls, weakening them over time. The small vessels (collaterals) in the Liver region become brittle and fragile, making them prone to rupture. Once bleeding starts, the Liver — already weakened — may not have the strength to store and regulate Blood effectively, leading to dangerous blood loss.

How Liver Qi Stagnation Leads to Bleeding in Cirrhosis or Variceal Rupture

In TCM, the Liver is responsible for ensuring the smooth flow of Qi throughout the body. When the Liver's Qi is blocked for a long time, it's like a busy city with constant traffic jams. This traffic in the Liver channels slows everything down, including Blood flow. Over the years, this stuck energy generates internal Heat, which irritates and inflames the Liver tissues and blood vessels.

This blockage also affects how fluids move in the body. Instead of flowing freely, fluids start to collect and mix with the Heat, creating a sticky, inflamed state known as Damp-Heat. This condition clogs up the Liver's network even more, increasing pressure inside the blood vessels and making the walls weaker.

As the years pass, poor circulation can progress into Blood Stasis, where Blood moves sluggishly and begins to pool. Think of it like traffic in a busy city: when cars crawl at a standstill for too long, exhaust and pressure build up. Over time, the roads (your blood vessels) begin to wear down, developing cracks and weak spots. In the Liver, this is like the tiny back roads — the collaterals — becoming worn and fragile, making them more prone to ruptures and bleeding.

When these weakened vessels finally give way, sudden bleeding can occur — sometimes into the intestines, sometimes into the esophagus — leading to the fresh red blood seen in severe cirrhosis or variceal rupture.

Different Individuals May Experience Different Symptoms From Cirrhosis or Variceal Bleeding

Bright Red Blood in Stool or Diarrhea. This is the hallmark sign. The stool may be loose, watery, or formed but streaked or mixed with fresh, bright red blood. The blood is often sudden in onset and may appear in large amounts during severe bleeding episodes.

Abdominal Swelling or Bloating. Cirrhosis often causes ascites — fluid buildup in the abdominal cavity — leading to visible swelling and a heavy sensation in the belly.

Jaundice. The skin and eyes may turn yellow due to the liver's reduced ability to process bilirubin.

Swelling in the Legs or Ankles. Fluid retention (edema) is common in advanced liver disease.

Dizziness, Lightheadedness, or Fainting. Significant blood loss can rapidly lower blood pressure and oxygen delivery, leading to these symptoms.

Paleness. Chronic or sudden blood loss can cause anemia, resulting in pale skin, lips, and nails.

Dark or Tea-Colored Urine. Caused by bilirubin buildup and possible dehydration.

Fatigue and Weakness. The liver's inability to filter toxins and the loss of blood can contribute to extreme tiredness.

Nausea or Loss of Appetite. Poor liver function often results in digestive discomfort and reduced desire to eat.

Visible Abdominal Veins. In advanced cirrhosis, engorged veins (caput medusae) may appear on the abdomen.

Confusion or Disorientation. In severe cases, toxins can build up in the blood and affect brain function, a condition known as hepatic encephalopathy.

Self Care and Support

Immediate Medical Attention. Variceal bleeding is a medical emergency. Any sudden appearance of bright red blood in stools or diarrhea in a person with known liver disease should be treated as urgent.

Medical Monitoring and Liver Support. Work closely with healthcare professionals to stabilize and support liver function, monitor cirrhosis progression, and track portal hypertension risk. Consistent follow-up appointments help adjust treatments as your condition changes.

Rest, Sleep, and Physical Activity. Prioritize early and restorative sleep — ideally from before 10 PM until around 7 AM — to align with the Liver's peak repair time in TCM and support overall healing.

Avoid straining, heavy lifting, or intense exercise that can increase portal vein pressure and trigger re-bleeding.

Maintain light, gentle movement like stretching, short walks, Tai Chi, or Qi Gong to promote circulation without overtaxing the body.

Dietary Strategies. Eat smaller, more frequent meals to ease digestive load and support Liver function. If anemic due to chronic bleeding, consume iron-rich foods like lean meats, black beans, and spinach, under medical supervision.

Hydration. Maintain good hydration to address dryness. Drink sufficient water and clear, non-caffeinated fluids. Consume cooling herbal teas or soups as advised by a TCM practitioner.

Herbal Support. Work with a qualified TCM practitioner for herbal remedies targeting Damp-Heat, bleeding disorders, and underlying Qi or Blood imbalances.

Emotional Well-being and Stress Reduction. In TCM, Liver Qi stagnation increases with emotional strain. Practice meditation, deep breathing, or gentle mind–body exercises to diffuse internal heat and improve emotional balance. Seek emotional support from friends, family, or counseling, as resolving emotional tension is key for Liver health.

Preventive Measures. Address underlying gastrointestinal issues, manage inflammation, and treat any infections to reduce recurrence risk.

Foods To Relieve Bleeding From Cirrhosis or Varices

Cooling fruits such as watermelon, cucumber, and pears can help reduce internal heat. However, because they are cold in nature, they should be consumed in moderation and ideally at room temperature or cooked, especially for those with Spleen Qi or Yang Deficiency, to avoid weakening digestive function.

Leafy greens, like spinach, Swiss chard, and bok choy, are cooling in nature and provide essential nutrients. To protect the Spleen and aid digestion, pair them with small amounts of warming ingredients such as ginger, garlic, or scallions when cooking.

Mung beans are known for their cooling properties in TCM and can help clear internal heat. You can prepare mung bean soup or porridge to cool the body, but to protect the Spleen and aid digestion, add a small amount of fresh ginger or dried tangerine peel during cooking.

Chinese yam (shan yao) is often used in TCM to nourish the Stomach and Spleen while addressing symptoms of heat. It can be added to soups or stews alongside mild warming herbs like goji berries or fresh ginger for better digestive balance.

Lotus root is considered a cooling food in TCM and can be used in various dishes to help alleviate heat-related symptoms. Cooking it with a few slices of ginger or stir-frying with scallions helps protect the Spleen and aid nutrient absorption.

Gelatin helps nourish and moisturize the body, making it a suitable option for addressing dryness. If used in desserts or drinks, pair it with warming spices like cinnamon or nutmeg to keep digestion strong.

Aloe vera is known for its cooling and soothing properties. Mix aloe vera gel into room-temperature herbal teas or blend with pear and a hint of ginger for a gentle, Spleen-friendly drink.

Porridge or congee is easily digestible and provides nourishment while being gentle on the digestive system. Use cooling ingredients such as mung beans or lotus seeds but cook with ginger or dried tangerine peel to harmonize the temperature nature. Every food has a temperature nature — not referring to how hot or cold the food is when served, but how it affects the body after digestion.

Coconut water is hydrating and can help combat dryness and dehydration associated with heat patterns. Drink it at room temperature and avoid excessive intake to prevent weakening the Spleen.

Herbs that help unblock Blood Stasis, stop bleeding, and relieve Liver congestion include Winged Euonymus Twig (Gui Jian Yu), Panax Notoginseng (San Qi), Red Peony Root (Chi Shao), and Cassia Twig (Gui Zhi). It is best to work with a qualified TCM practitioner when using herbal formulas. For daily support, herbal teas such as chrysanthemum tea can provide a cooling effect on the body. To balance its cool nature, brew with a small piece of dried tangerine peel or a few goji berries to add warmth and support to the Spleen.

Foods That Can Worsen Bleeding From Cirrhosis or Varices

Spicy and warming foods, such as chili peppers, curry, and other heat-inducing spices, can increase internal heat and inflammation. Avoid these in your diet.

Alcohol consumption can worsen heat patterns in the body and exacerbate bleeding issues. It's best to avoid alcohol in this condition.

Caffeine is considered heating in TCM and can add excessive heat in the body. Coffee and caffeinated beverages should be avoided in this condition.

Fried and greasy foods can be difficult to digest and may aggravate digestive problems, contributing to heat and dryness. Opt for lighter cooking methods.

Processed and spicy snacks, particularly those with added flavoring and preservatives, can be heating and irritating to the digestive system.

Excessive sugar intake can lead to dampness and heat in the body. Minimize the consumption of sugary foods and beverages.

Red meat, particularly when cooked in spicy or greasy dishes, can exacerbate heat patterns. Consider leaner and lighter protein sources.

High salt intake can lead to fluid retention and contribute to dampness. Reducing salt intake is advisable.

Dairy can worsen symptoms in some individuals with strong heat patterns. In general, even those with healthy digestion may find that regular consumption of dairy weakens their system over time.

Smoking can introduce heat into the body and worsen underlying conditions. Quitting smoking can be a beneficial step.

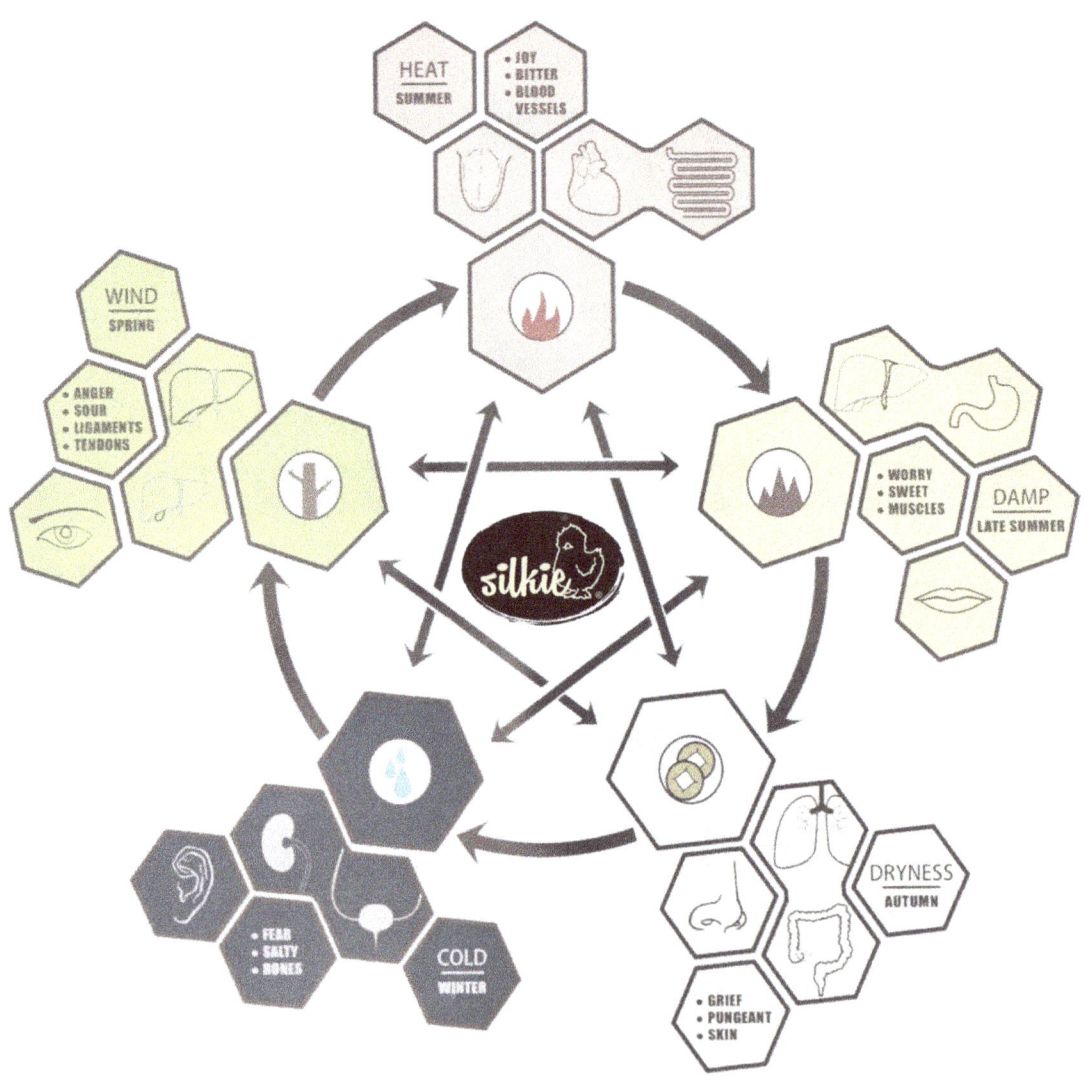

Exploring Fecal Incontinence Causes

Fecal incontinence, or the inability to control the passing of stool, can manifest in different ways. Sometimes, it means a sudden, overwhelming urge to defecate with no time to make it to the toilet. Other times, stool might leak without any prior sensation or warning. Understanding the underlying causes is key to addressing this challenging condition.

Western Medical Perspectives on Fecal Incontinence

From a Western medical standpoint, fecal incontinence often boils down to issues with the muscles or nerves involved in bowel control, or problems with stool consistency. Diarrhea can overwhelm the anal sphincter's ability to hold stool, especially if it's severe or sudden. Conversely, constipation can also play a role. When stool becomes hard and impacted, liquid stool can leak around it, leading to incontinence. Damage to the muscles of the pelvic floor or anal sphincter, perhaps from childbirth, surgery, or injury, can weaken their ability to hold stool. Similarly, nerve damage — from conditions like diabetes, stroke, spinal cord injury, or multiple sclerosis — can disrupt the signals between the brain and the rectum, preventing proper control.

Fecal Incontinence Through the Lens of Traditional Chinese Medicine

Traditional Chinese Medicine offers a different perspective on the causes of fecal incontinence, often linking it to specific patterns of internal imbalance.

One acute pattern is Damp-Heat Toxin in the colon, which can arise during severe viral infections, similar to conditions with very high fever. This intense internal Heat and Dampness can spread quickly throughout the body, overwhelming the system and causing widespread body aches, dizziness, restlessness, and, in extreme cases, fainting. In TCM, when Heat becomes excessive, it can disturb the Heart and agitate the Shen (the mind/spirit), which explains why mental clarity and consciousness may be affected. Meanwhile, the colon's function is severely disrupted, leading to uncontrolled bowel movements, sometimes with mucus and blood. Treatment focuses on cooling the body, draining Heat and Dampness, protecting the digestive tract, and calming the Heart to restore balance.

For more chronic forms of fecal incontinence, TCM often points to Spleen and Kidney Yang Deficiency or Sinking Qi due to Spleen Deficiency. These conditions develop over time and reflect a lack of foundational energy within the body:

- **Spleen and Kidney Yang Deficiency:** This pattern is frequently associated with chronic diarrhea, particularly occurring around 5 AM (the "colon time" in the body's natural clock). The Spleen's "Yang" energy is crucial for warmth and strength in the digestive system, while the Kidneys' "Yang" energy is vital for warmth in the lower body and maintaining overall body control. When both are deficient, it leads to persistent diarrhea, uncontrollable bowel movements, weak legs, and cold extremities.

- **Spleen Yang Deficiency:** The Spleen in TCM is responsible for transforming and transporting food and fluids. A deficiency in Spleen Yang impairs digestion and nutrient transport, resulting in loose or watery stools and a general inability to properly hold things in.

- **Kidney Yang Deficiency:** The Kidneys are seen as the root of the body's foundational energy. When Kidney Yang is weak, it can lead to a loss of control over the lower body, including the anal sphincter, contributing to issues like chronic diarrhea and incontinence.

- **Sinking Qi Due to Spleen Deficiency:** In TCM, Spleen Qi (energy) plays a crucial role in "holding things in place" and maintaining the upward direction of bodily functions. If the Spleen's Qi is weak, it can "sink," leading to feelings of pressure or heaviness in the anus, and even conditions like anal prolapse, hernia, directly impacting bowel control.

Understanding these diverse causes, from both Western and TCM perspectives, is crucial for effective diagnosis and developing a comprehensive treatment plan for fecal incontinence.

Understanding the Different Types of Constipation and What Causes Them

Constipation, a common and often uncomfortable issue, is characterized by infrequent or hard and dry bowel movements. Understanding its diverse causes, from both conventional Western medicine and Traditional Chinese Medicine perspectives, is crucial for effective management and prevention.

Western Medical Causes of Constipation

From a Western medical standpoint, lifestyle choices and physiological factors are often at the root of constipation. A primary culprit is an insufficient intake of dietary fiber. Fiber is essential because it adds bulk to stool and helps retain water, making it softer and easier to pass. Fruits, vegetables, whole grains, and beans are excellent sources. Closely related is inadequate hydration; when you don't drink enough water, stools become dry and difficult to move through the intestines. While the "eight glasses a day" rule is common, individual needs vary based on factors like activity level, climate, and health conditions, so listening to your body's thirst cues is key.

Beyond diet and hydration, certain external factors can contribute. Many medications, including some pain relievers, antidepressants, and antipsychotics, list constipation as a common side effect. A lack of physical activity also slows down the digestive system, making regular bowel movements less likely; incorporating at least 30 minutes of moderate exercise most days of the week can be beneficial. Physiological changes like pregnancy can lead to constipation as the expanding uterus puts pressure on the rectum. Finally, underlying medical conditions such as hypothyroidism and diabetes can disrupt normal bowel function and lead to chronic constipation.

Traditional Chinese Medicine Perspectives on Constipation

In addition to lifestyle choices and physiology, Traditional Chinese Medicine attributes the causes of constipation to imbalances of Heat, Qi, Yin, and Yang. These patterns of imbalances provide a deeper understanding of individual presentations:

Excess Heat in the Stomach and Intestines: This pattern manifests with classic constipation symptoms like dry, hard stools, often accompanied by abdominal discomfort, a red face, dry mouth, and bad breath. This imbalance is frequently linked to dietary choices, particularly excessive consumption of spicy foods, and lifestyle factors like late-night activities that can generate internal heat.

Qi Stagnation: When the body's Qi (vital energy) isn't flowing smoothly, it can lead to constipation. Individuals with Qi stagnation might experience stools that are soft or hard, but consistently struggle with straining during bowel movements and a feeling of incomplete evacuation. Excessive gas is also common. Emotionally, chronic stress is a significant contributor to Qi stagnation, highlighting the mind-body connection in TCM.

Yang Deficiency: This pattern indicates a lack of warmth and vital energy, particularly in the Spleen and Kidneys. Symptoms extend beyond the digestive tract to include cold limbs (hands and feet), often alongside hard or soft stools, hiccups, and generalized abdominal discomfort. This pattern is frequently observed in older individuals or in those whose lifestyle gradually depletes the body's Yang energy. Over time, habits such as excessive sexual activity, frequent alcohol consumption, overeating rich or greasy foods, lack of physical activity, or staying up late into the night can weaken the Kidneys and Spleen. These behaviors, combined with prolonged stress or poor self-care, chip away at the body's fundamental warmth, leaving it unable to generate sufficient energy to support healthy digestion and circulation.

Blood and Yin Deficiency: Constipation stemming from a deficiency in Blood and Yin points to a lack of nourishing fluids and substances needed to lubricate the intestines and moisten the stool. This results in difficulty expelling stools and a profound feeling of fatigue after bowel movements, as the body struggles to complete the digestive process without adequate resources.

By considering both Western and TCM perspectives, a more comprehensive understanding of constipation emerges, paving the way for targeted and effective management strategies.

Who's Most Susceptible to Constipation?

Constipation is a pervasive issue that can significantly diminish comfort and quality of life. While many factors can contribute to this digestive roadblock, certain demographics and lifestyle choices make some individuals more prone to constipation.

Vulnerable Populations: Seniors and Women

As we age, our bodies undergo natural changes that can make us more susceptible to constipation. For seniors, the digestive system itself can become less efficient. The muscles lining the intestines may weaken, and the nerves responsible for coordinating bowel movements can become less responsive. This leads to a slower transit time of stool, allowing more water to be absorbed and resulting in harder, drier stools. Furthermore, older adults are often on multiple medications, some of which have constipation as a common side effect. Reduced mobility, decreased fluid intake due to a diminished thirst sensation, and changes in dietary habits also play a significant role, creating a perfect storm for constipation.

Women, throughout their lives, face unique physiological challenges that elevate their risk. Hormonal fluctuations are a major factor; changes in estrogen and progesterone during menstruation, pregnancy, and menopause can directly impact gut motility, slowing down the passage of food through the digestive tract. During pregnancy, the expanding uterus can physically press against the rectum, making it harder for stool to pass, while hormonal shifts also contribute. Blood loss during menstruation and childbirth, from a Traditional Chinese Medicine perspective, can lead to a "Blood Deficiency," which can indirectly contribute to constipation by failing to adequately lubricate the intestines. Women also, on average, have longer colons than men, which means stool has a greater distance to travel, allowing more water to be absorbed and making stools firmer.

Lifestyle and Behavioral Contributors

Beyond inherent biological factors, our daily habits and emotional states profoundly influence bowel regularity. A sedentary lifestyle is a prime example. When we spend prolonged periods sitting or are generally inactive, our digestive system tends to slow down. Physical movement helps stimulate the natural muscular contractions of the intestines (peristalsis) that push stool along. Without this gentle "prodding," bowel function can become sluggish, leading to stool accumulation and hardening.

The profound connection between our gut and our brain means that high stress can directly contribute to constipation. When the body perceives stress, it activates the "fight or flight" response, diverting resources away from "non-essential" functions like digestion. Stress hormones, such as cortisol and epinephrine, can slow down intestinal movement. Chronic stress, in particular, can disrupt the delicate balance of the gut microbiome and interfere with the nerve signals that regulate bowel function, effectively "tying the gut in knots."

Finally, seemingly simple poor bowel habits can surprisingly perpetuate constipation. Ignoring the urge to have a bowel movement, perhaps due to busyness, public restroom aversion, or simply habit, is a common culprit. When the urge is ignored, the stool sits in the rectum longer, allowing more water to be reabsorbed, making it harder and more difficult to pass later. Irregular bowel habits also disrupt the body's natural "schedule," making it harder for the colon to establish a consistent rhythm for defecation. Over time, this can lead to a reduced sensitivity to the urge itself, creating a vicious cycle of infrequent and difficult bowel movements.

Self-Care and Support

- **Cultivate regular defecation habits.** Establish a consistent routine for bowel movements by going at the same time daily. Start your morning with warm water or honey water to help stimulate bowel movement. Apple cider vinegar is okay, however daily consumption can lead to excessive acidity that impacts Stomach function.

- **Moderate exercise** relieves stress and increases bowel movements.

- **Abdominal massage,** clockwise around the navel, stimulates bowel peristalsis.

Foods That Affect Bowel Movements

- **Unripe bananas** contain tannins that hinder digestion. Ripe bananas with soluble fiber are a better choice.

- **Fried foods** are high in fat and can slow digestion. Opt for high-fiber options instead.

- **Processed foods** are low in fiber and high in fat, sugar, and salt. Processed foods can contribute to constipation. Choose whole, unprocessed foods.

- **Red meat** takes longer to digest due to its high fat and protein content. Lean protein sources like chicken or fish are better options.

- **Dairy** can be difficult to digest due to its low fiber and high fat and protein content. For some individuals, this heaviness slows down digestion and can lead to constipation, especially when consumed in excess or alongside other rich foods. On the other hand, for those who are lactose sensitive or intolerant, dairy often causes diarrhea. This happens because the body lacks sufficient lactase, the enzyme needed to break down lactose, leading to fermentation in the intestines, bloating, cramps, and loose stools. In TCM, dairy is considered damp-forming, which can either block the bowels and cause constipation or overwhelm the digestive system and trigger diarrhea, depending on the person's underlying pattern.

- **Coffee and tea** with caffeine can reduce water retention, but they can also lead to dehydration, resulting in dry and hard stools.

Foods That Improve Constipation

- **Prunes and prune juice** are high in cellulose, so they soften stools and ease the passage.

- **Beans** are rich in dietary fiber so they promote digestion when fully cooked.

- **Whole-grain products** increase stool weight and stimulate peristalsis when prepared well.

- **High-fiber foods** such as fruits, vegetables, and whole grains can help relieve constipation by increasing stool bulk and promoting bowel movement. However, in TCM, raw and overly sweet fruits are considered cooling and Dampness-forming, which can weaken the Spleen and slow digestion, especially in those with Spleen Qi or Yang Deficiency. For these individuals, fiber-rich foods are best consumed cooked and served warm to protect digestive function.

- **Adequate hydration** keeps stools soft and reduces their hardness.

- **Healthy fats** help lubricate the intestines and ease stool passage. Nuts such as almonds, cashews, and walnuts — or oils like sesame, olive, and flaxseed — can facilitate smoother bowel movements when eaten in moderation.

- **Fruits rich in natural enzymes,** like papaya, pineapple, and kiwi, can be enjoyed as a snack to enhance digestion due to their rich natural enzyme content.

- **Yogurt.** In Western nutrition, yogurt is valued for its probiotics, which can aid digestion and sometimes relieve constipation. However, in Traditional Chinese Medicine (TCM), yogurt is still considered a dairy product, and all dairy is thought to be cold and Dampness-forming in nature. Its cooling and moistening qualities may weaken the Spleen, particularly in those with Spleen Qi or Yang Deficiency. While it may offer short-term relief by softening stools, over time it can aggravate Dampness and lead to more serious digestive imbalances.

Herbal bone broths or even plain bone broths can support digestion and help relieve certain types of constipation in TCM

Constipation from Blood Deficiency or Yin Deficiency. In TCM, Blood moistens the intestines. When there's a deficiency, stools can become dry and hard, and bowel movements infrequent. Bone broth is rich in collagen, minerals, and essence (Jing), which help nourish Blood and Yin, indirectly moistening the intestines. Especially useful for postpartum women, elderly people, or those recovering from illness.

Constipation from Qi Deficiency. When Qi is weak, the "pushing force" for bowel movement is reduced, leading to sluggish stools even if they're not extremely dry. Bone broth strengthens Spleen and Stomach Qi, improving digestion and bowel motility.

Constipation from Cold in the Intestines. Warm bone broth supports Yang and warms the digestive system, which can help in cases where coldness is slowing intestinal movement. Particularly good if the person also has cold hands/feet, prefers warmth, and feels better with warm drinks.

Constipation is due to Excess Heat or Damp-Heat in the intestines. Traditional bone broth, especially from marrow bones, is warming, rich, and tonifying — which can aggravate Heat and Damp-Heat. Adding cooling vegetables (like winter melon, bitter melon, celery, cucumber, chrysanthemum greens) offsets this warming nature. Using lean meat instead of fatty cuts reduces greasiness, which is important because Damp-Heat thrives in rich, oily environments.

Lactose Intolerance in Traditional Chinese Medicine

The following section is written by Catherine Yung, who shares both her personal experience with lactose intolerance and the Traditional Chinese Medicine perspective. This is one of several contributions she has made to this book, where her writings weave together lived experience and TCM wisdom to make each topic relatable and clear.

Have you ever felt a tummy ache after having milk or cheese? That could be because your body has a hard time breaking down something called "lactose." Lactose is a sugar found in milk, and when your body can't break it down, it can make your tummy feel upset. In Traditional Chinese Medicine, we explain this in a slightly different way.

In TCM, your body has an energy called "Qi" (say it like "chee"), which helps keep you strong and healthy. Your Stomach and Spleen work together to turn the food you eat into energy so you can run, play, and grow! But when your Stomach and Spleen are not working well, especially with foods like milk or cheese, it can lead to what we call "dampness." Dampness is like when something gets too wet and heavy, like your clothes after being caught in the rain. When your Stomach and Spleen can't handle dairy, it creates too much Dampness, making your tummy feel uncomfortable and upset. This is what we call lactose intolerance.

When your body doesn't have enough of a special helper called lactase, which is supposed to break down lactose, it can cause all sorts of tummy troubles. You might feel bloated, like there's too much air in your tummy. You might need to run to the bathroom quickly, or even have runny poop (diarrhea). Your tummy might even make funny grumbling noises. In TCM, this is seen as your Stomach and Spleen struggling to deal with the Dampness caused by the dairy.

Let me tell you about my own experience with lactose intolerance. I used to have a lot of tummy problems whenever I had dairy. My poop would get very loose and runny, and I'd have to rush to the bathroom, sometimes more than once! I remember once after drinking milk tea, I had to go to the restroom three times in a row — and it felt like my stomach was doing flips. It was uncomfortable and even embarrassing.

I also used to have trouble eating pizza with cheese or anything with dairy in it. Pizza was the worst. I loved pizza, but I had to peel the cheese off every slice just so I wouldn't feel sick. But it didn't always help. My stomach still felt funny, and sometimes I had to lie down because the cramps were too much. I'd get gassy, my tummy would make whale noises, and sometimes I'd have to rush to the bathroom before finishing my slice! My poop would be all soft and runny, and I felt so uncomfortable. It wasn't fun at all. I always had to ask for food without cheese or say no to ice cream, which made me sad. But after I started taking TCM allergy formula along with formulas that support the Spleen, I noticed a big change. My tummy calmed down, the bathroom trips slowed down, and — hooray! — I could eat pizza again once in a while with the cheese on! Even a little ice cream here and there doesn't scare me anymore. It's such a relief to be able to eat some of my favorite foods again and not worry about what might happen afterward.

When you have lactose intolerance, TCM doctors might suggest some things to help your tummy feel better. For example:

Eat warm, cooked foods that are easy to digest, like soups and stews.

Avoid dairy products like milk and cheese until your tummy feels stronger.

Drink special herbal teas or formulas that can help strengthen your Stomach and Spleen.

So if milk or cheese ever makes your tummy hurt, don't worry! It's just your body's way of saying it needs a little help. With some simple changes and some TCM support, your stomach can feel much better, and you'll be back to enjoying your favorite foods again!

TCM Perspective on Common Gut Health Practices & Mistakes

In Traditional Chinese Medicine, gut health depends on the harmony of the Spleen and Stomach Qi. While many modern health practices aim to improve digestion, they often overlook TCM principles — and in some cases, may unintentionally weaken digestion over time.

Many people turn to fiber supplements like Metamucil to regulate digestion. While fiber is beneficial, TCM cautions against excessive intake of raw or cold fiber, as it can burden the Spleen Qi, leading to bloating and sluggish digestion. Warm, cooked fiber sources — such as steamed vegetables, congee, millet, or cooked pears — are gentler and better support Spleen function.

Probiotic-rich foods like yogurt, kefir, and kimchi are widely promoted for gut health, but in TCM, they have drawbacks. Yogurt and kefir are dairy-based and can be hard to digest. Additionally, flavored yogurt and kefir have added sugar which contributes to the formation of dampness in the body. Kimchi is sour in flavor and cold in nature, especially since it's often eaten chilled — both qualities can irritate the stomach lining, generate Dampness, and weaken Spleen Qi if consumed excessively. The key is moderation, balancing them with warming foods like ginger tea or cooked rice porridge to offset their cooling or damp-producing effects. Fermented foods like kombucha, pickles, and tempeh are also recommended in modern wellness circles, but their cold and sometimes overly sour nature can further weaken digestion in those with Spleen Qi Deficiency. Small amounts may be helpful, but only when balanced with warming herbs and cooked foods.

Probiotic supplements are another common choice, but in TCM, simply adding probiotics does not address deeper imbalances — such as Spleen Qi Deficiency or Liver Qi Stagnation — that may be causing poor digestion in the first place. Additionally, both probiotic and prebiotic supplements often require preservatives for shelf stability, and even capsule or tablet forms (including so-called "vegetable capsules") must use chemical binders to hold their structure. These additives may irritate sensitive digestive systems and are rarely addressed in mainstream probiotic discussions. Concentrated probiotics can also overwhelm a weak digestive system rather than gradually strengthening it. Prebiotic foods like garlic, onions, bananas, and asparagus can help nourish beneficial bacteria, but raw prebiotics may be too cold or pungent, disturbing digestion in sensitive individuals. Light cooking improves digestibility and prevents excessive cooling of the gut.

Another popular trend is intermittent fasting. While short-term fasting can reduce food stagnation and support metabolism, TCM warns that prolonged or repeated fasting can weaken Spleen and Stomach Qi — especially in individuals prone to weak digestion. Over time, extreme fasting can lead to Blood and Qi Deficiency, with symptoms like fatigue, dizziness, hair loss, poor concentration, and a pale complexion. Fasting can also reduce nutrient intake, increasing the risk of malnourishment. Many people feel lighter and more energized during a fast, but this often happens because the digestive system is temporarily relieved of its workload — not because the root imbalance is resolved. Once regular eating resumes, the original digestive issues typically return. If fasting continues without addressing the underlying cause, it can further deplete the body's vital resources. TCM instead favors a balanced approach — warm, easily digestible meals eaten at regular times to nourish Qi and Blood while preventing food stagnation.

Some people turn to enemas for constipation relief. While they can provide temporary improvement, overuse may weaken Qi and Yang, creating dependency. A more sustainable approach is to include moistening foods such as sesame oil, cooked pears, honey, and steamed leafy greens, alongside lifestyle practices that support healthy bowel movements.

Gut-healing supplements like L-glutamine, collagen, and digestive enzymes are often used to repair the intestinal lining. While beneficial in some cases, TCM emphasizes that true digestive healing comes from whole, warm, nourishing foods like bone broth with cooked vegetables, congee, and lightly seasoned soups, rather than relying solely on supplements.

Ultimately, TCM teaches that gut health is not one-size-fits-all. Overconsumption of raw, cold, or overly fibrous foods can weaken digestion instead of strengthening it. Excessive reliance on supplements — without addressing diet, lifestyle, and underlying imbalances — often provides only temporary relief. Long-term digestive health comes from balance, warmth, and nourishment, guided by your own constitution and seasonal needs. Warm fluids, herbal teas, and gentle cooking methods protect Spleen Qi and support healthy, resilient digestion far better than extreme or trendy approaches.

Diet and Lifestyle Tips for Healthy Bowel Movements

In this chapter, we'll delve into practical strategies you can implement to promote healthy bowel movements and overall digestive wellness. Your daily choices regarding food and lifestyle can have a profound impact on the state of your digestive system.

Hydration. Start your day with a cup of warm water to cleanse your system before breakfast. Drink an adequate amount of water throughout the day. Proper hydration helps keep your stools soft and facilitates their passage.

Food Variety. In your daily diet include different fruits, grains, vegetables, meats, nuts, or eggs. Avoid repeating the same ingredients frequently. To avoid malnutrition or vitamin deficiency.

Meal Timing. Maintain a regular eating schedule with three meals at regular times (around 8 a.m., 12 p.m., and 5 p.m.) to establish a dependable routine for your digestive system. Consistency can promote regular bowel movements.

Meals Portions. Breakfast is the medium portion; Lunch is the biggest portion; Dinner is the smallest portion, it's better to eat slightly less to prevent strain on your digestive system.

Mindful Eating. Practice mindful eating by chewing your food slowly and thoroughly. This aids in the digestion process and can prevent overeating.

Early Dinner. Allow at least 2 ½ to 3 hours between your last meal of the day, to avoid going to sleep with a full stomach.

Fiber-Rich Diet. Increase your fiber intake by incorporating more fruits, vegetables, whole grains, and legumes into your meals. Fiber adds bulk to your stool, making it easier to pass.

Stress Management. Implement stress-reduction techniques like deep breathing exercises, meditation, or yoga. Reducing stress can alleviate digestive problems.

Physical Activity. Include regular physical activity in your routine, as it can help stimulate your digestive system and promote regular bowel movements.

Balanced Yin–Yang Meal. A well-balanced meal should avoid creating excess Heat or Cold in the digestive system, allowing food to be transformed and absorbed more efficiently. For example, a typical balanced meal might include a combination of meat, vegetables, and grains. Occasionally incorporating small amounts of probiotic-rich foods, such as kefir or sauerkraut, can also support the gut microbiome. However, in TCM, these foods are often cooling in nature, so they are best enjoyed in moderation rather than as a daily staple.

Processed Foods. Reduce your consumption of processed foods, sugary snacks, and unhealthy fats. These can lead to digestive issues.

Medication Management. If you're on medication, be aware of any potential digestive side effects and discuss them with your healthcare provider.

Body Awareness. Healthy digestion isn't just about what you eat, but also about how you respond to your body's natural signals. Pay attention to the urge to have a bowel movement and try not to delay it, as ignoring the signal can lead to constipation or irregular habits. When you do go, avoid straining — forcing puts unnecessary pressure on the intestines and can weaken digestive function over time.

By implementing these practical tips and making informed choices regarding your diet and lifestyle, you can support a healthy digestive system and enjoy the benefits of regular, comfortable bowel movements.

Seeking Professional Guidance

In this chapter, we'll discuss the importance of seeking professional guidance when it comes to your digestive health. While understanding your bowel movements and implementing healthy habits is crucial, there are times when consulting a healthcare provider is necessary.

When to See a Healthcare Provider

Persistent Digestive Issues: If you experience persistent digestive problems such as chronic constipation, diarrhea, abdominal pain, or blood in your stool, it's essential to consult a healthcare provider. These symptoms could be signs of underlying conditions that require diagnosis and treatment.

Sudden Changes: If your bowel habits suddenly change without an obvious reason, seek medical attention. Sudden and unexplained shifts in bowel movements can indicate a health issue that needs evaluation.

Family History: If you have a family history of digestive diseases or colon cancer, it's crucial to discuss screening and preventive measures with a healthcare provider.

Age and Risk Factors: Age can be a risk factor for certain digestive conditions. Regular screenings and check-ups become more critical as you age to detect any issues early.

Persistent Pain: If you experience persistent abdominal pain or discomfort, especially if it worsens or interferes with your daily life, consult a healthcare provider for evaluation.

Screening and Diagnosis

Healthcare providers may recommend various diagnostic tests and screenings to assess your digestive health. These may include:

Colonoscopy: A procedure to examine the colon for signs of colorectal cancer and other digestive conditions.

Endoscopy: An examination of the upper digestive tract using a flexible tube with a camera.

Blood Tests: To check for markers of digestive conditions and nutrient deficiencies.

Imaging: Such as X-rays or CT scans to visualize the digestive organs.

Stool Analysis: To detect infections, blood in the stool, or other abnormalities.

Treatment and Management

Based on the diagnosis, your healthcare provider will develop a personalized treatment plan. Treatment may involve lifestyle changes, dietary adjustments, or herbal supplements depending on the condition.

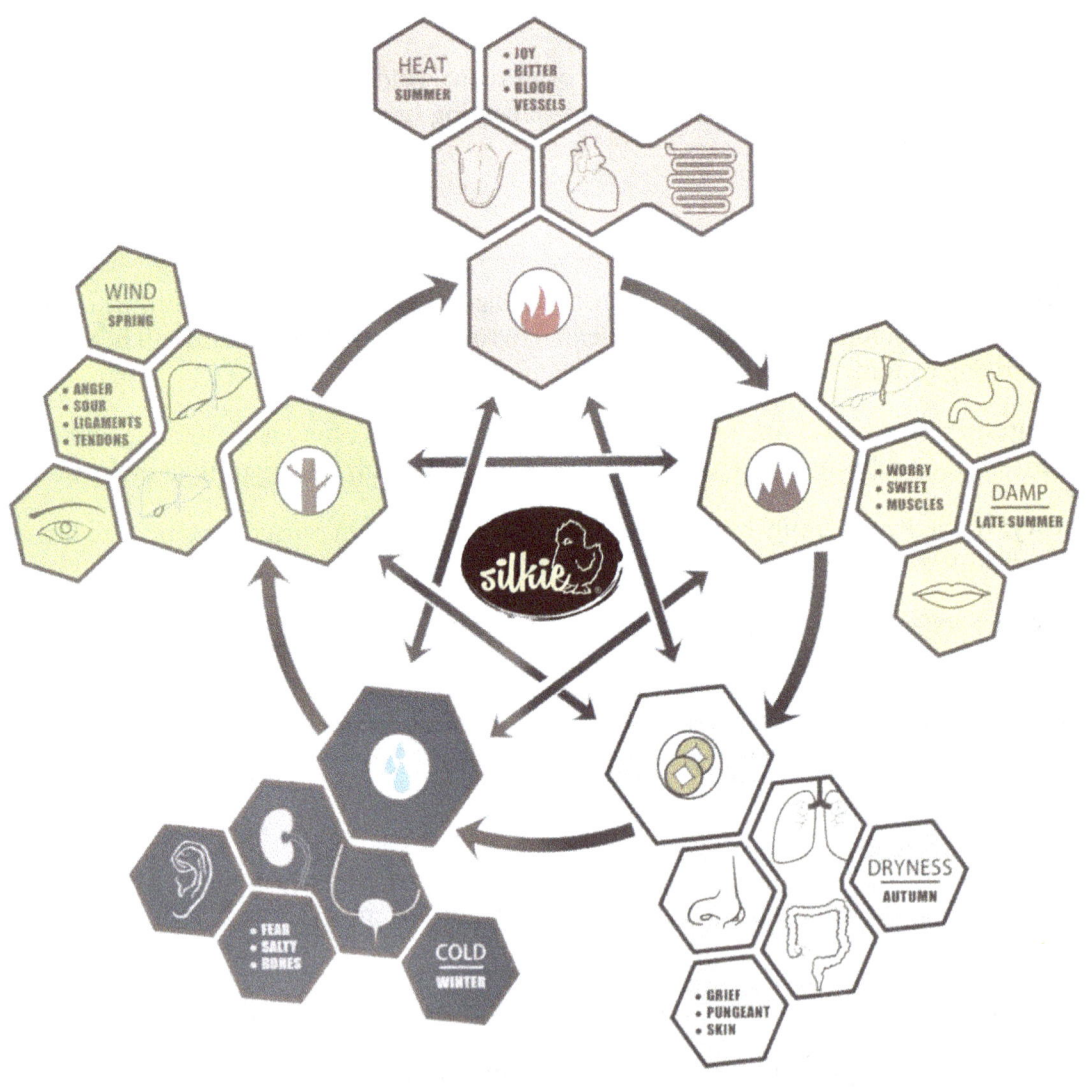

Conclusion: Your Poop, Your Health Story

If there's one thing this book has shown, it's that poop is never "just poop." In Traditional Chinese Medicine, it is a direct reflection of your internal balance — a daily progress report written by your body in a language that, once understood, can guide you toward better health. The color, shape, smell, texture, and frequency of your stools are all telling you something about the state of your Qi, Blood, Yin, Yang, and organ systems.

Throughout these pages, you've learned how to recognize patterns — from Spleen Qi Deficiency to Intestinal Damp-Heat, from Blood Stasis to Liver Qi Stagnation — and how diet, lifestyle, and Chinese medicine can restore harmony. You've also seen how certain patterns may be early warning signs for deeper health issues, giving you the chance to take action before they become more serious.

But the real power lies in what you do next. Knowing the signs is only the first step. Acting on them — by adjusting your meals to match your constitution, seeking professional guidance when symptoms persist, and making lifestyle changes that protect your digestive health — is how you turn knowledge into healing.

Remember:

Your poop changes because your body changes. Seasons shift, stress levels rise and fall, and your diet and habits evolve over time. This means your stools will also change — sometimes subtly, sometimes dramatically. That's why observation is not a one-time effort but an ongoing conversation with your body.

If you take away only one thing from this book, let it be this: your bathroom breaks are an opportunity to check in with your health every single day. You don't need fancy equipment or complicated tests — just your own awareness, a little TCM knowledge, and the willingness to listen to what your body is saying.

The next time you look into the toilet bowl, you're not just seeing waste — you're seeing the footprints of your health journey. And now, you have the tools to read them.

So, trust your gut — literally — and let your poop guide you toward a healthier, more balanced, and more vibrant life.

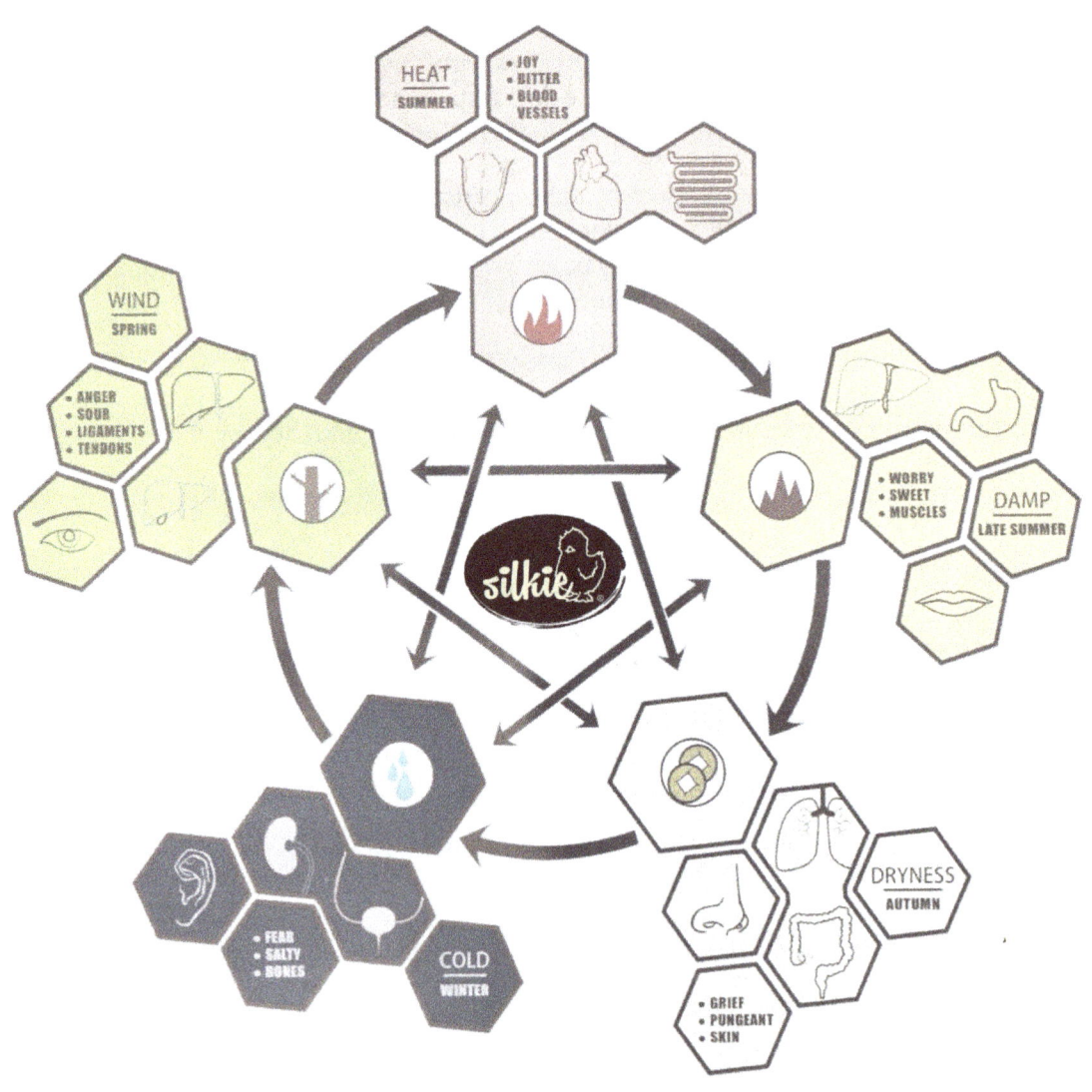

TCM Digestive Pattern Quick Guide

Digestive Conditions & TCM Meanings

Condition	Possible TCM Pattern	What It Means	Suggested Actions	Page
Fecal Incontinence	Spleen & Kidney Yang Deficiency	Weak organ Qi fails to control bowels, leakage	Warm foods, Yang tonics, strengthen Spleen & Kidney	p.131
	Spleen Yang Deficiency	Cold digestion, sluggish bowels, leakage	Cooked meals, avoid raw/cold foods	p.131
	Kidney Yang Deficiency	Cold limbs, urinary issues, poor control	Tonify Kidney Yang with warming herbs, bone broth	p.132
	Sinking Qi (Spleen Deficiency)	Prolapse, sagging organs, leakage	Strengthen Spleen Qi, avoid overwork, gentle exercise	p.132
Constipation	Excess Heat in Stomach/Intestines	Dry, hard stools, red face, bad breath	Clear Heat, hydrate, avoid spicy/fried foods	p.133
	Qi Stagnation	Straining, incomplete evacuation, stress-related	Relieve stress, move Qi (citrus peel, breathing, walking)	p.133
	Yang Deficiency	Cold limbs, sluggish bowels, weak digestion	Warm meals, Yang tonics, avoid raw/cold foods	p.133
	Blood & Yin Deficiency	Dry stools, fatigue after movement	Nourish Blood & Yin (dang gui, sesame, pears, soups)	p.134
Lactose Intolerance	Spleen Qi Deficiency with Dampness	Dairy creates Dampness → bloating, loose stools, runny poop	Avoid dairy, strengthen Spleen, herbal support, warm soups	p.137

Stool Types & TCM Meanings

Stool Appearance	Possible TCM Pattern	What It Means	Suggested Actions	Page
Bumpy/lumpy stool	Kidney Deficiency, long-term Qi and Fluid Deficiency	Elderly, weak Kidney Qi, fatigue, back pain	Tonify Kidney Qi/Yin with black beans, sesame, mushrooms	p.25
Dry, cracked stool	Internal Heat and Dryness in the Intestines, Fluid Deficiency	Excess heat burns fluids, drying stool	Avoid spicy/fried foods; add cooling foods (melon, cucumber)	p.33
Dry-hard then soft stool	Spleen Qi Deficiency with Dampness	Weak Spleen unable to fully transform food	Eat warm, cooked meals, tonify Spleen Qi	p.37
Finger-like stool	Malnutrition, Liver Qi Stagnation affecting Spleen, Qi Deficiency	Weak digestion, insufficient nourishment	Balanced meals, blood tonics	p.43
Fluffy, mushy stool	Liver & Spleen Disharmony	Stress injures digestion, food not transformed	Manage stress, avoid greasy foods	p.51
White dots/worms stool	Parasites, weak Spleen function	Dampness, poor gut defense	Deworming herbs, hygiene, avoid raw meats	p.57
Soft blobs with straining stool	Early Stage of Qi & Blood Deficiency, Spleen Qi Deficiency	Not enough strength to push stool	Tonify Qi & Blood, soups & tonics	p.63
Floating stool	Spleen Qi Deficiency without Dampness, Poor Fat Digestion	Poor absorption of nutrients	Warm cooked meals, avoid dairy/greasy foods	p.71
Sink and sticky stool	Dampness blocking the Spleen	Incomplete digestion, mucus formation, greasy/heavy stools	Avoid dairy, fried foods, sweets; drink warm teas; strengthen Spleen Qi	p.77
Dry, hard, dark Pebbles stool	Blood Dryness, Stagnation in Large Intestine, prolonged Qi & Blood Deficiency	Chronic lack of fluids & Blood	Nourish Blood with dates, sesame, Dang Gui	p.81
Dark/light watery stool	Food retention or poisoning	Acute toxic diarrhea	Flush toxins with mung bean, soup, rest, hydrate	p.87
Dark yellow watery stool	Heat & Dampness in Stomach/Spleen	Foul-smelling diarrhea with inflammation	Avoid spicy/fried foods, herbs to clear Damp-Heat	p.93
Light yellow watery stool	Cold-Damp in Stomach/Spleen	Fishy-smelling diarrhea with cold injures digestion	Warm cooked meals, ginger tea	p.97
Green stool	Liver Qi Stagnation, Stomach/Spleen Deficiency with Coldness, Damp-Heat in Intestines	Stress or poor digestion of greens	Exercise, soothe Liver Qi with teas	p.103
Pale stool	Gallbladder/Liver Qi Issues, Spleen Yang Deficiency	Weak bile flow	Support Liver/Gallbladder, avoid greasy foods	p.107
Bloody stool with mucus/pus stool	Intestinal Damp-Heat with bleeding	Inflammation + blood in intestines	Clear Damp-Heat, avoid greasy/spicy	p.113
Black stool	Blood Stasis, upper digestive bleeding	Oxidized blood from stomach/duodenum	Emergency care; TCM cool Blood, clear Heat	p.119
Fresh red bloody stool	Liver disease, variceal bleeding	Severe urgent condition	Emergency care	p.125

Food & Poop Matching Guide

Foods That Support Healthy Poop

Food	Positive Stool Effect	TCM Benefit	Best Use
Sesame seeds, black sesame	Softens hard stools	Nourishes Blood & Yin	Sprinkle on rice or porridge
Honey	Moistens dryness, eases constipation	Lubricates Intestines	Warm water + honey in the morning
Pears & apples	Softer, smooth stools	Moistens Lung & Intestines	Eat cooked/poached in cool months
Sweet potatoes, yams	Balanced, well-formed stools	Strengthens Spleen Qi	Steam or bake, not fried
Rice porridge (congee)	Gentle, easy stools	Strengthens digestion, clears Dampness	Great breakfast option
Mung beans	Clears toxic diarrhea	Clears Heat & Toxin	Make mung bean soup in summer
Bone broth	Builds strong digestion, firmer stools	Nourishes Qi & Blood	Sip warm, avoid excess salt

Foods That Can Cause Imbalance

Food	Common Stool Effect	TCM Explanation	Balance Tip
Dairy (milk, cheese, ice cream)	Loose, sticky stools, bloating	Creates Dampness → weakens Spleen	Replace with bone broth or warm soups; add ginger tea
Spicy foods (chili, hotpot, peppers)	Dry, cracked, burning stools	Generates Internal Heat → dries fluids	Balance with cooling foods (cucumber, pear)
Fried foods (fries, fried chicken, chips)	Sticky, smelly stools; floating stools	Damp-Heat accumulation in Spleen/Stomach	Bake/steam instead of frying; add bitter greens
Red meat (beef, lamb, pork)	Hard, difficult-to-pass stools	Heavy to digest, increases Stagnation & Heat	Pair with vegetables, eat smaller portions
Cold/raw foods (salads, fruits, smoothies, sushi)	Loose watery stools, abdominal discomfort	Injures Spleen Yang → creates Cold-Damp	Eat cooked vegetables, soups, stews instead
Excess sugar/sweets	Loose stools, sticky or smelly stools	Creates Phlegm & Dampness	Replace with fruit in moderation; use honey or dates
Alcohol & coffee	Loose, urgent stools, dehydration	Disperses fluids, damages Qi, causes Heat & Damp	Drink warm teas or water; limit daily intake

TCM Stool Types & Herbs Guide

Poop Flow Chart: From Stool to Solution

Look at Your Stool Type and Identify Pattern → Silkie Formulas. A plus sign (+) indicates combining formulas together. A comma (,) between formulas indicates optional choices.

If Stool is Hard/Dry

Dry, cracked stool → *Internal Heat* → Heartburn Formula (for dry/hard stools with reflux, bloating, discomfort) and/or Constipation Formula (for sluggish bowels with straining) + Kidney Yin (for dryness, night sweats, hot sensations) + Spleen Support (Fluid Stagnation from improper digestion or Spleen Qi Deficiency), Allergy Formula (for weak digestion that can lead to sensitivities and food triggers), Immune (for Qi Deficiency, low resistance)

Dry-hard then soft stool → *Spleen Qi Deficiency + Dampness* → Spleen Support (for bloating, fatigue, weak digestion) + Intestinal Support (alternating constipation/diarrhea) and/or Heartburn Formula (for dry-hard stools with epigastric discomfort), Allergy Formula (for dampness, sensitivities), Immune (for Qi Deficiency, low resistance)

Dry, dark pebbles → *Blood Dryness* → Blood and Stamina (for fatigue, pale complexion, blood deficiency) + Kidney Yin (for nourishing fluids) + Spleen Support (for weak digestion) + Heartburn (for constipation with upper digestive discomfort), Allergy Formula (for dampness, food triggers), Immune (for Qi Deficiency, low resistance)

If Stool is Soft/Loose

Fluffy, mushy stool → *Liver & Spleen Disharmony* → Spleen Support (for weak Spleen Qi) + Stomach Support (heat) (for diarrhea from spicy/greasy food) and/or Stomach Support (cold) (for dairy/raw food-related loose stools), Allergy Formula (for weak digestion that can lead to sensitivities and dampness), Immune (for Qi Deficiency, low resistance)

Soft blobs, straining → *Qi & Blood Deficiency* → *Blood Dryness* → Blood and Stamina (for fatigue, pale complexion, blood deficiency) + Kidney Yin (for nourishing fluids) + Spleen Support (for weak digestion) + Heartburn (for weak digestion & Liver Qi Stagnation), Allergy Formula (for weak digestion that can lead to sensitivities and dampness), Immune (for Qi Deficiency, low resistance)

Floating stool → *Spleen Qi Deficiency ± Dampness* → Spleen Support (to strengthen Qi and absorb nutrients) + Heartburn (to support digestion & Qi circulation), Allergy Formula (for weak digestion that can lead to sensitivities and dampness), Immune (for Qi Deficiency, low resistance)

Sinking & sticky stool → *Dampness Blocking Spleen* → Stomach Support (cold) (for dairy/raw food-related loose stools) and/or Stomach Support (heat) (for greasy/spicy food-related loose stools) + Spleen Support (to strengthen Qi and absorb nutrients) + Heartburn (to support digestion & Qi circulation), Allergy Formula (for weak digestion that can lead to sensitivities and dampness), Immune (for Qi Deficiency, low resistance)

If Stool is Watery/Diarrhea

Watery diarrhea (dark to light) → *Food Retention or Toxic Heat* → Intestinal Support (for acute food retention/poisoning) and/or Stomach Support (heat) (for foul, hot diarrhea) + Kidney Yin (to restore fluids) + Spleen Support (to strengthen Qi and absorb nutrients) + Chronic Diarrhea (for midnight pooping, long-term loose stools), Allergy Formula (for weak digestion that can lead to sensitivities and dampness), Immune (for Qi Deficiency, low resistance)

Dark yellow watery stool → *Heat & Dampness in Stomach/Spleen* → Stomach Support (heat) (for heat diarrhea) and/or Heartburn (for upper GI discomfort) + Spleen Support (to strengthen Qi and absorb nutrients) + Kidney Yin (to restore fluids), Chronic Diarrhea (if long-term or midnight pooping), Allergy Formula (for weak digestion that can lead to sensitivities and dampness), Immune (for Qi Deficiency, low resistance)

Light yellow watery stool → *Cold-Damp in Stomach/Spleen* → Stomach Support (cold)(for dairy/raw food-related diarrhea), Chronic Diarrhea (midnight pooping, chronic watery diarrhea), Allergy Formula (for weak digestion that can lead to sensitivities and dampness), Immune (for Qi Deficiency, low resistance)

If Stool is Bloody/Discolored

Green stool → *Liver Qi Stagnation* → Mood (for emotional stress) + Heartburn Formula (for Liver Qi stagnation), Spleen Support (to strengthen Qi and absorb nutrients), Stomach Support (heat) (for greasy/spicy food-related loose stools), Allergy Formula (for weak digestion that can lead to sensitivities and food triggers), Immune (for Qi Deficiency, low resistance)

Pale stool → *Liver/Gallbladder Qi Issues* → Detox Liver (for sluggish bile flow) + Spleen Support (to strengthen Qi and absorb nutrients) + Heartburn Formula (for Liver Qi stagnation) + Blood and Stamina (for Blood Deficiency & fatigue) + Lower Body Block (for stagnation, lower GI blockage), Allergy Formula (for weak digestion that can lead to sensitivities and food triggers), Immune (for Qi Deficiency, low resistance)

Bloody stool + mucus/pus → *Intestinal Damp-Heat* → Hemorrhoid (for bleeding vessels) + Intestinal Support (alternating constipation/diarrhea) + Spleen Support (to strengthen Qi and absorb nutrients) + Blood and Stamina (to replenish deficiency from blood loss), Allergy Formula (for weak digestion that can lead to sensitivities and food triggers), Immune (for Qi Deficiency, low resistance)

Black stool → *Blood Stasis / Bleeding* → Emergency + Silkie support like Blood and Stamina (to replenish deficiency from blood loss) + Heartburn (for upper GI discomfort) + Spleen Support (to strengthen Qi and absorb nutrients), Allergy Formula (for weak digestion that can lead to sensitivities and food triggers), Immune (for Qi Deficiency, low resistance)

Fresh red bloody stool → *Varices/Liver Disease* → Emergency + Silkie support like Blood and Stamina (to replenish deficiency from blood loss) + Spleen Support (to strengthen Qi and absorb nutrients) + Lower Body Block (for stagnation, lower GI blockage) + Intestinal Support (for intestinal bleeding, alternating constipation/diarrhea), Detox Liver (for liver Qi stagnation, sluggish bile flow, toxic heat in the liver), Hepatitis (for chronic liver inflammation, supporting healthy liver function and detoxification), Allergy Formula (for weak digestion that can lead to sensitivities and food triggers), Immune (for Qi Deficiency, low resistance)

Special Cases

Bumpy/lumpy stool → *Kidney Deficiency* → Kidney Yin (for cooling fluids, dryness, night sweats, hot sensations) and/or Kidney Yang (for warming metabolism, cold limbs, backache, fatigue), Heartburn Formula (for Liver Qi stagnation), Spleen Support (to strengthen Qi and absorb nutrients), Allergy Formula (for weak digestion that can lead to sensitivities and dampness), Immune (for Qi Deficiency, low resistance)

Finger-like stool → *Malnutrition, Qi/Blood Deficiency* → Blood and Stamina (for Blood Deficiency & fatigue) + Energy Endurance (builds Qi & Blood for nourishment) + Spleen Support (to strengthen Qi and absorb nutrients) + Heartburn (for fatigue, weak digestion), Allergy Formula (for weak digestion that can lead to sensitivities and food triggers), Immune (for Qi Deficiency, low resistance)

White dots/parasites → *Parasite Infestation* → Parasite Formula (for worms, parasites); consult TCM practitioner

Lactose intolerance symptoms → *Spleen Qi Deficiency w/ Dampness* → Allergy Formula (for weak digestion that can lead to sensitivities and food triggers) + Immune (for Qi Deficiency, low resistance) + Spleen Support (to strengthen Qi and absorb nutrients) + Heartburn Formula (for Liver Qi stagnation)

Incontinence → *Kidney & Spleen Yang Deficiency / Sinking Qi* → Kidney Yang (for warming metabolism, cold limbs, backache, fatigue) + Spleen Support (to strengthen Qi and absorb nutrients) + Blood and Stamina (for Blood Deficiency & fatigue), Allergy Formula (for weak digestion that can lead to sensitivities and food triggers), Immune (for Qi Deficiency, low resistance)

Why Allergy Formula & Immune Booster Appear in Every Category

In today's world, allergies are far more common than in the past. Food sensitivities, seasonal allergies, and environmental triggers (like pollen, dust, and chemicals) often overlap with digestive imbalances. At the same time, modern lifestyles — filled with stress, overwork, and poor diet — weaken the immune system and make the body more reactive.

A lot of people think allergies are no big deal until they flare up with rashes, sneezing, itchy eyes, or a runny nose. Many turn to over-the-counter allergy drugs, which often only mask symptoms temporarily. Over time, these reactions can worsen, forcing people to cut out more foods while still developing new sensitivities. This cycle not only disrupts digestion but also creates nutrient imbalances that weaken the body even further.

From a TCM perspective, these factors create extra burdens of Dampness, Qi Deficiency, and Heat, all of which worsen digestive problems. The Immune formula works by strengthening Wei Qi, the body's protective shield that guards against external pathogens and allergens. Together with the Allergy Formula, these remedies reduce flare-ups, support nutrient absorption, and help the body stay resilient.

Other formulas may also be helpful depending on your specific needs. Energy Endurance is recommended if you often experience physical fatigue or low stamina, giving your body the support it needs to feel more energized. If you find yourself struggling with mental fatigue or frequent brain fog, the Focus Formula can provide clarity and concentration. For those showing signs of Blood Deficiency, such as a pale complexion, dizziness, heavy fatigue, or weak stools, Blood and Stamina can be especially beneficial in replenishing and strengthening the body.

Clinical Story:

One patient came to me after years of taking antihistamines for "minor allergies." At first, she only had itchy eyes and sneezing, but soon she started reacting to more foods, including dairy and wheat. Weather changes would also set her off — a cool breeze or sudden seasonal shift triggered sneezing, watery eyes, nasal itching, or even hives. By the time she sought help, her digestion was weak — she often had loose stools, bloating, and fatigue. After starting the Allergy Formula and Immune Booster, along with gentle dietary changes, she noticed her stools became more formed, her energy steadier, and her reactions less frequent. What seemed like "just allergies" had actually been undermining her digestion for years. Supporting her Wei Qi and Spleen together broke the cycle.

Because of this, both formulas are included across stool types as supportive options. Even if the root cause is not directly allergy- or immunity-related, they help protect against future triggers and maintain overall balance.

Silkie Herbal Formulas & Stool Types

Stool Type / Symptom	Pattern in TCM	Recommended Silkie Formula(s) Use "+" to combine formulas together "," to indicate optional choices.
Dry, cracked stool	Internal Heat	Heartburn and/or Constipation + Kidney Yin + Spleen Support, Allergy, Immune
Dry-hard then soft stool	Spleen Qi Deficiency w/ Dampness	Spleen Support + Intestinal Support and/or Heartburn, Allergy Formula, Immune
Dry, hard, dark pebbles	Blood Dryness (Qi/Blood Deficiency)	Blood and Stamina + Kidney Yin + Spleen Support + Heartburn, Allergy Formula, Immune
Fluffy, mushy stool	Liver & Spleen Disharmony	Spleen Support + Stomach Support (heat) and/or Stomach Support (cold), Allergy Formula, Immune
Soft blobs requiring straining	Qi & Blood Deficiency	Energy Endurance + Kidney Yin + Spleen Support + Heartburn, Allergy Formula, Immune
Floating stool	Spleen Qi Deficiency without Dampness	Spleen Support, Heartburn, Allergy Formula, Immune
Sink and sticky stool	Dampness blocking Spleen	Stomach Support (cold) and/or Stomach Support (heat) + Spleen Support + Heartburn
Watery stools (dark or light)	Food Retention, Toxic Damp-Heat	Intestinal Support and/or Stomach Support (heat) + Kidney Yin + Spleen Support + Chronic Diarrhea, Allergy Formula, Immune
Dark yellow watery stool	Damp-Heat in Stomach/ Spleen	Stomach Support (heat) and/or Heartburn + Spleen Support + Kidney Yin, Chronic Diarrhea, Allergy Formula, Immune
Light yellow watery stool	Cold-Damp in Stomach/ Spleen	Stomach Support (cold), Chronic Diarrhea, Allergy Formula, Immune
Green stool	Liver Qi Stagnation, Damp-Heat	Mood + Heartburn, Spleen Support, Stomach Support (heat), Allergy Formula, Immune
Pale stool	Liver/Gallbladder Qi Deficiency	Detox Liver + Spleen Support + Heartburn + Blood and Stamina + Lower Body Black, Allergy Formula, Immune
Bloody stool with mucus/pus	Intestinal Damp-Heat with bleeding	Hemorrhoid + Intestinal Support + Spleen Support + Blood and Stamina, Allergy Formula, Immune
Black stool	Blood Stasis / Upper GI Bleeding	Blood and Stamina + Heartburn + Spleen Support, Allergy Formula, Immune
Fresh red bloody stool	Advanced Liver disease / Varices	Blood and Stamina + Spleen Support + Lower Body Block + Intestasis, Detox Liver, Hepatitis, Allergy Formula, Immune
Bumpy/lumpy stool	Kidney Deficiency	Kidney Yin and/or Kidney Yang, Allergy Formula, Immune
Finger-like stool	Malnutrition, Qi & Blood Deficiency	Blood and Stamina + Energy Endurance + Spleen Support + Heartburn, Allergy Formula, Immune
White dots/parasites stool	Parasite Infestation	Parasite Formula, Allergy, Immune; consult TCM practitioner
Lactose intolerance	Spleen Qi Deficiency w/ Dampness	Allergy Formula + Spleen Support + Immune Booster
Incontinence (chronic leakage)	Spleen/Kidney Yang Deficiency, Sinking Qi	Kidney Yang + Spleen Support + Blood and Stamina, Chronic Diarrhea, Allergy Formula, Immune

Stool Types & Herbal Support in TCM

Stool Type	TCM Pattern	Suggested Herbs / Formulas	Notes
Bumpy/lumpy stool	Kidney Deficiency	Rehmannia (Shu Di Huang), Cornelian Cherry (Shan Zhu Yu), Gordon Euryale Seed (Qian Shi)	Nourish Kidney Yin & Qi, support lower back & bones
Dry, cracked stool	Internal Heat	Scutellaria Root (Huang Qin), Ophiopogon (Mai Men Dong), Rhubarb (Da Huang)	Clears Heat, moistens dryness
Dry-hard then soft stool	Spleen Qi Deficiency w/ Dampness	Codonopsis (Dang Shen), Poria (Fu Ling), Atractylodes (Bai Zhu), Tangerine Peel (Chen Pi)	Strengthens Spleen, improves transformation of food
Finger-like stool	Malnutrition, Qi/Blood Deficiency	Angelica Root (Dang Gui), Codonopsis Root (Dang Shen), Goji Berries (Gou Qi Zi)	Nourishes Blood, boosts Qi, supports digestion
Fluffy, mushy stool	Liver & Spleen Disharmony	Bupleurum Root (Chai Hu), White Peony Root (Bai Shao), Poria (Fu Ling)	Smooths Liver Qi, strengthens Spleen
White dots/worms	Parasites	Smoked Plum (Wu Mei), Chinaberry Tree Bark (Ku Lian Pi), Areca Seed (Bing Lang)	Expels parasites, antimicrobial properties
Soft blobs, straining	Qi & Blood Deficiency	Codonopsis (Dang Shen), Angelica Root (Dang Gui), Rehmannia Root (Shu Di Huang)	Tonifies Qi & Blood, builds energy for elimination
Floating stool	Spleen Qi Deficiency ± Dampness	Shan Yao (Chinese Yam), Poria (Fu Ling), Chen Pi (Tangerine Peel), Atractylodes (Bai Zhu)	Strengthens Spleen Qi, transforms Damp
Sink & sticky stool	Dampness blocking Spleen	Poria (Fu Ling), Atractylodes (Bai Zhu), Magnolia Bark (Hou Po), Agastache (Huo Xiang)	Expels Dampness, improves digestion
Dry, hard, dark pebbles	Blood Dryness (Qi/Blood Deficiency)	Sheng Di Huang (Rehmannia), Hei Zhi Ma (Black Sesame), Huo Ma Ren (Hemp Seed)	Nourishes Yin & Blood, moistens Intestines
Dark/light watery stool	Food retention / poisoning	Mung Beans, Hawthorn Fruit (Shan Zha), Raphanus Seed (Lai Fu Zi)	Clears toxins, drains Damp-Heat
Dark yellow watery stool	Heat & Dampness in Stomach/Spleen	Scutellaria Root (Huang Qin), Phellodendron Bark (Huang Bai), Gardenia Fruit (Zhi Zi)	Clears Damp-Heat, relieves diarrhea
Light yellow watery stool	Cold-Damp in Stomach/Spleen	Dried Ginger (Gan Jiang), Atractylodes (Cang Zhu), Poria (Fu Ling), Magnolia Bark (Hou Po)	Warms Yang, expels Cold
Green stool	Liver Qi Stagnation w/ Damp-Heat	Bupleurum Root (Chai Hu), Gentian Root (Long Dan Cao), Capillaris (Yin Chen Hao)	Smooths Liver Qi, clears Heat
Pale stool	Gallbladder/Liver Qi Issues	Curcuma Root (Yu Jin), Bupleurum Root (Chai Hu), Capillary Wormwood (Yin Chen Hao)	Promotes bile flow, regulates Liver Qi
Bloody stool + mucus/pus	Intestinal Damp-Heat	Scute (Huang Qin), Angelica Tails (Dang Gui Wei), and Fructus Sophorae (Huai Hua)	Clears Damp-Heat, cools Blood
Black stool	Blood Stasis / upper GI bleeding	Codonopsis (Dang Shen), Angelica Root (Dang Gui), Notoginseng root (Tianqi)	Cools Blood, stops bleeding (urgent Western care too)
Fresh red bloody stool	Severe Liver disease / Varices	Winged Euonymus Twig (Gui Jian Yu), Red Peony Root (Chi Shao), Panax Notoginseng (San Qi)	Stops bleeding, but urgent Western care is priority

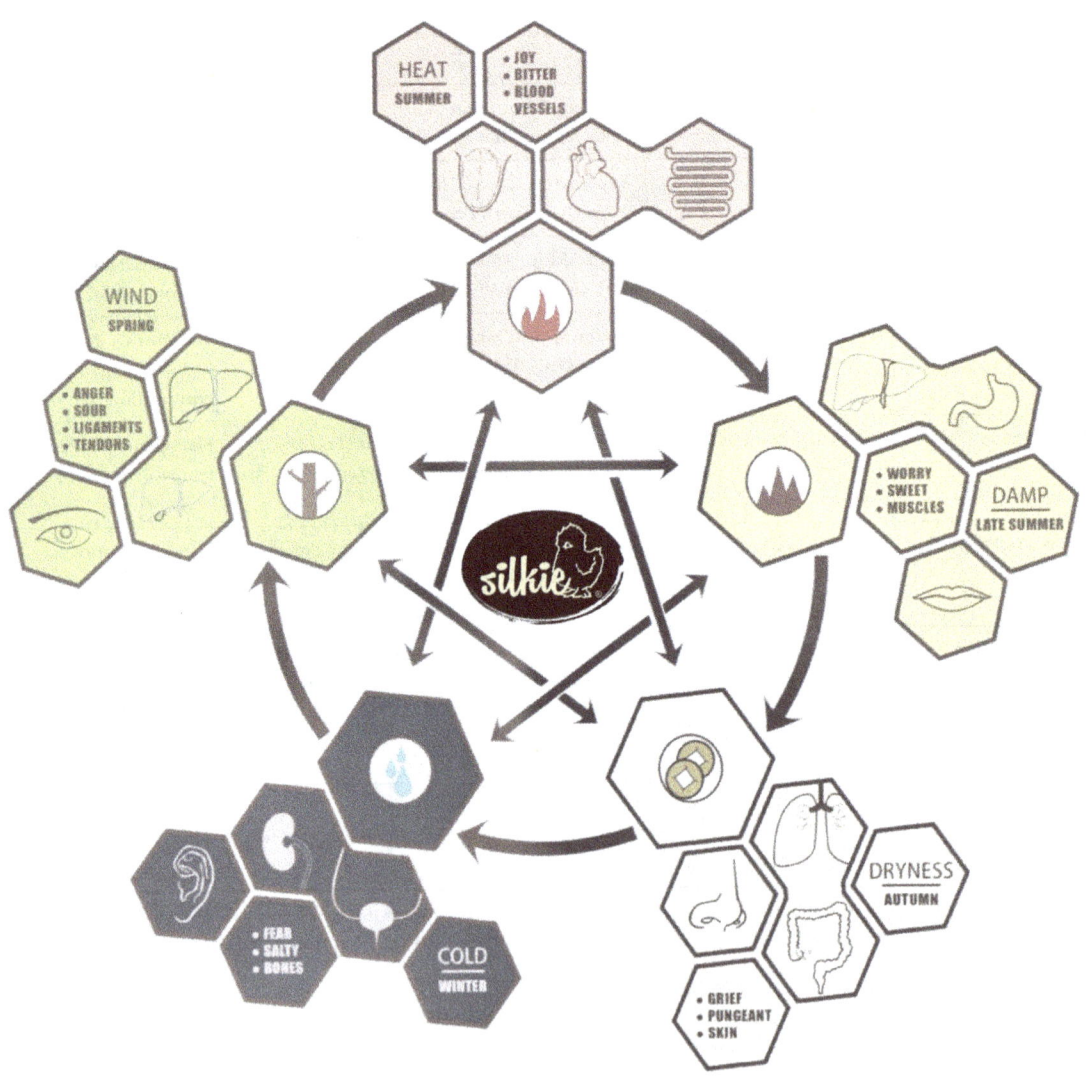

Stool Tracker

Weekly Reflection Questions

At the end of each week, reflect on your log.

Did your stool change with certain foods?

Did stress, sleep, or emotions affect digestion?

Were there days you felt more energetic vs. sluggish?

Did any red-flag symptoms appear (blood, black stool, sudden diarrhea)?

Daily Stool Log

Date	Time	Stool Type (shape/texture)	Color	Odor	Ease of Passing	Food Eaten Before	Emotions / Stress Level	Notes
Example: Jan 10	7:15 AM	Soft blobs, straining	Light brown	Mild	Took effort	Pizza, soda	mild	Felt bloated

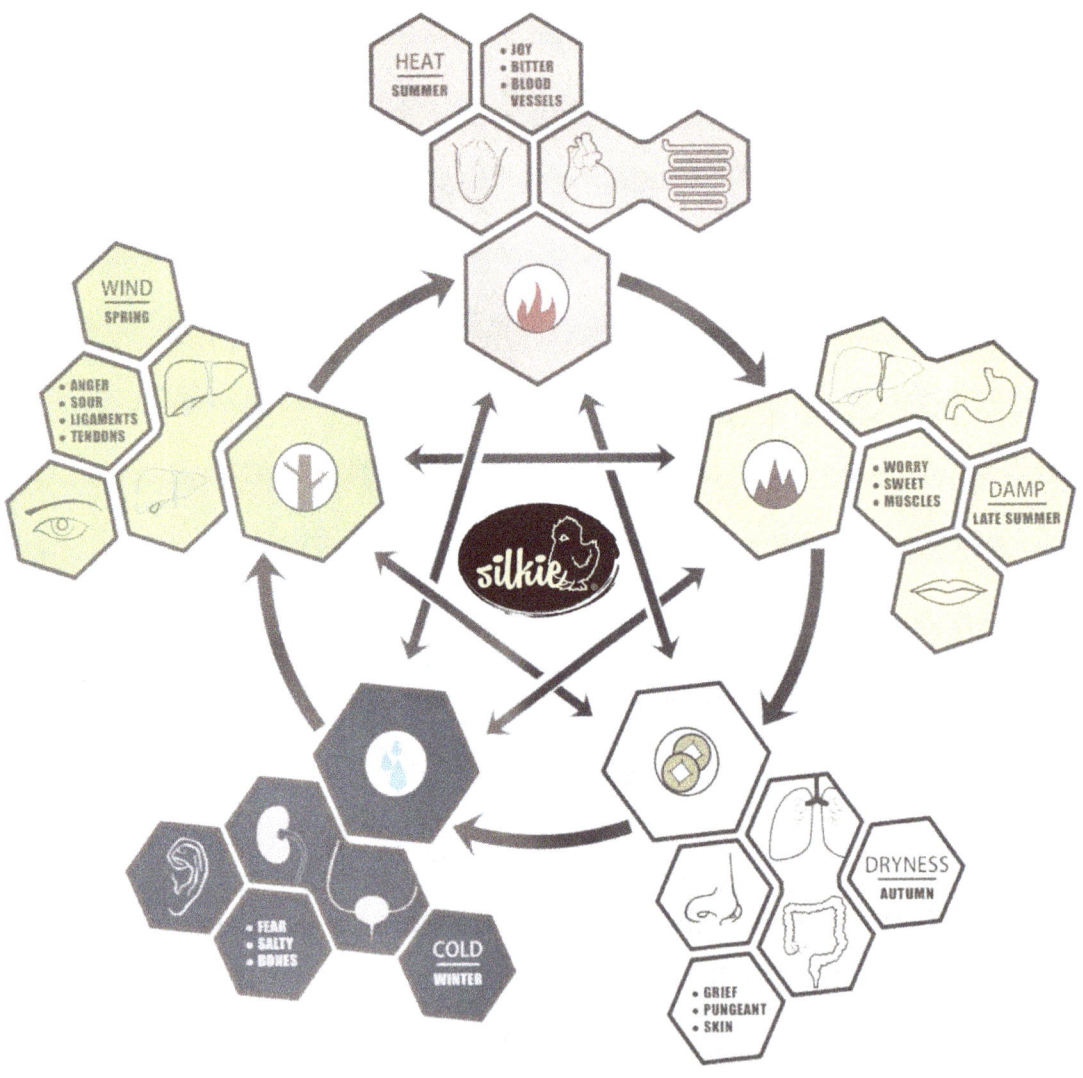

Index

A
Abdominal cramps or pains — p. 28, 35, 46, 53, 59, 94, 99, 104, 115, 122
Abdominal discomfort — p. 28, 35, 39, 67, 72, 78, 82, 89, 104, 109, 115
Abdominal discomfort or pain or fullness after eat — p. 39, 78, 94
Abdominal discomfort is relieved after a bowel movement — p. 53
Abdominal sensitive to pressure — p. 35
Abdominal swelling (fluid build up) — p. 39, 127
Acid reflux — p. 53, 89
Acne — p. 35
Allergic reactions — p. 53, 59
Anal (itching, irritation, pain or discomfort) — p. 53, 59
Anemia — p. 46, 53, 122, 127
Appetite changes (excessive hunger, Stomach Heat) — p. 53, 94
Appetite changes (poor appetite, Spleen Qi Deficiency) — p. 53

B
Bad breath — p. 35, 79, 89
Belching — p. 53, 67, 82, 89, 109
Bile lack of (pale stools, Gallbladder) — p. 107
Bile too much (green stools, Liver) — p. 103
Bitter taste in the mouth — p. 35, 53, 79, 92, 104, 122
Black stool — p. 22, 119
Bloating — p. 35, 39, 53, 59, 67, 72, 82, 89, 99, 104, 109
Blood in stool bright red (hemorrhoids, Liver Heat, variceal bleeding) — p. 21, 23, 113, 125
Blood in stool black tar-like (upper digestive bleeding) — p. 119
Blood Deficiency (dry stools, Qi and Blood Deficiency, constipation) — p. 63, 81
Bloody diarrhea — p. 115, 127
Blurred vision — p. 83
Brain Fog — p. 28, 45, 67, 72, 78
Bright red blood — p. 21, 23, 113, 125
Brittle hair — p. 45, 82
Brittle nail — p. 45, 83
Brittle bone — p. 46
Brown stool — p. 11, 16
Bruising and easy bleeding — p. 39
Bumpy/lumpy stool (Kidney Deficiency) — p. 25
Burping — p. 53, 67, 82, 89, 109

C
Changes in Blood Pressure — p. 46
Changes in Heart Rate — p. 46
Cold-Damp stools (light yellow, fishy odor) — p. 97
Cold extremities (hands or feet) — p. 73, 83, 122
Cold sensation — p. 28, 39, 109

Colon health (peristalsis, bowel movement timing) — p. 4, 7-9
Confusion or disorientation — p. 127
Congestion — p. 72, 78
Constipation — p. 29, 35, 46, 89, 133, 134
Constipation from Blood and Yin Deficiency, Yang Deficiency (pebble-like stool) — p. 26, 133, 134
Constipation from heat (dry, cracked stool) — p. 33, 133
Constipation from Qi Stagnation (straining) — p. 63, 133
Cough — p. 59, 72
Cracks in stool (Internal Heat, Dryness) — p. 33

D

Dairy (Dampness, Phlegm, lactose intolerance) — p. 137
Damp-Heat (foul odor, sticky stool, diarrhea) — p. 87, 93
Dampness (mucus stools, bloating, heaviness) — p. 77
Dark yellow urine or tea-colored urine — p. 35, 84, 93, 105, 127
Dark stools (bleeding vs. excess Heat) — p. 33, 119
Dark to like watery stool multiple times a day — p. 87
Dark yellow stool or watery stool — p. 17, 93
Decreased libido — p. 28
Delayed wound healing — p. 46, 66
Diarrhea acute toxic (food poisoning, Damp-Heat) — p. 87
Diarrhea chronic loose stools in the middle of the night (Spleen Yang Deficiency) — p. 107
Diarrhea cold-Damp diarrhea (fishy odor, light yellow to clear water) — p. 97
Diarrhea heat-Damp diarrhea (yellow, foul) — p. 93
Diarrhea lactose-related (Spleen Qi weakness, Dampness) — p. 137-138
Different color of stools — p. 15-23
Difficulty concentrating — p. 28, 45, 59, 67, 72, 78, 83
Difficulty falling asleep or staying asleep — p. 48, 53, 67, 83, 105, 110
Dizziness — p. 45, 67, 83, 122, 127
Dry, cracked stool (Internal Heat) — p. 33
Dry hair — p. 61, 73, 82
Dry, hard, dark pebbles that are hard to pass stool — p. 81
Dry-hard then soft stool (Spleen Qi Deficiency with Dampness) — p. 37
Dry (mouth, throat, skin or eye) — p. 29, 35, 45, 67, 82, 83
Dry stools (Blood Dryness) — p. 81
Dry stools (Heat in the Stomach and Intestines) — p. 33
Dry stools (Yin Deficiency) — p. 25

E

Early-morning diarrhea — p. 109
Easy bruising — p. 39
Edema — p. 28, 39, 46, 72, 78, 95, 127
Emotional symptoms (anger) — p. 83, 95
Emotional symptoms (anxiety) — p. 28, 35, 53, 59, 83
Emotional symptoms (depression) — p. 28, 46, 83
Emotional symptoms (fear) — p. 28
Emotional symptoms (frustration) p. 53
Emotional symptoms (instability) — p. 53, 73, 109
Emotional symptoms (irritability) — p. 28, 35, 53, 59, 73, 95, 104, 109
Emotional symptoms (mood swing) — p. 53, 73, 104, 109
Emotional symptoms (nervousness) — p. 28
Emotional symptoms (overthinking, worry) — p. 73, 83
Emotional symptoms (restlessness) — p. 53, 59
Emotional symptoms (sadness) — p. 46, 83
Emotional symptoms (stress) — p. 46, 53

Energy (role in digestion, stool formation) — p. 3-5
Enuresis while sleeping (can not hold the urine) — p. 28
Enuresis during the day (can not hold the urine) — p. 28
Excessive vaginal discharge — p. 39
Excessive heat or heat in the blood — p. 122
Excessive phlegm or mucus — p. 39, 72
Eye issues — p. 97, 105, 110

F
Fainting — p. 127
Fatigue — p. 28, 39, 45, 53, 59, 67, 72, 78, 82, 89, 94, 105, 110, 115, 122, 127
Fecal incontinence (Spleen/Kidney Yang Deficiency, Heat toxin) — p. 131, 132
Feel hot (palms, soles or chest) — p. 29
Feeling of coldness — p. 88
Fertility problems — p. 35, 39, 46
Fever (low-grade fever) — p. 53, 59, 105, 115
Finger-thin stool (malnutrition, Spleen Qi Deficiency) — p. 43
Floating stools (Spleen Qi Deficiency, Dampness) — p. 71
Fluffy/mushy stools (Liver Qi stagnation, Spleen Deficiency) — p. 51
Frequent bowel movememts — p. 87, 93, 97, 104, 109
Frequent illnesses and infection — p. 67
Frequent urinary infections — p. 28, 31
Frequent urination — p. 28, 35, 40
Foods cause imbalance chart — p. 150
Foods support healthy poop chart — p. 149
Forgetfulness — p. 72, 78, 83
Fullness after meals — p. 72
Fullness in the abdomen — p. 39, 94
Fullness in the chest and side of ribs — p. 53, 67
Fullness in the chest and upper abdomen — p. 53, 73, 82, 99

G
Gallbladder (pale stool, bile obstruction) — p. 107
Gastritis — p. 46
Gas — p. 46, 57, 59, 69
Gastrointestinal disorders — p. 46, 59
Green stool (Liver Qi stagnation, Damp-Heat in Liver/Gallbladder) — p. 18, 103
Greasy or difficult-to-flush stool — p. 72
Gut health practices (overuse of probiotics, laxatives, cold smoothies) — p. 139, 140

H
Hair brittle — p. 45
Hair loss — p. 45
Headache — p. 93, 97, 105, 110
Heartburn — p. 79
Heat sensations — p. 29, 35
Heaviness — p. 78, 94, 99, 104
Heavy Limbs — p. 72
Herbs Guide (Spleen tonics, Dampness-resolving, Heat-clearing, Yin nourishing) — p. 151-155
Hives — p. 59
Hormonal Imbalances — p. 46
Hot flashes — p. 29
Hydration (stool softness, Qi and Fluid balance) — p. 136

I
IBS (constipation or diarrhea) — p. 43, 63, 115
Impaired cognitive function — p. 28

Impaired growth — p. 46
Impaired nutrient absorption — p. 46
Impotence or infertility — p. 28, 35, 39, 42
Incontinence (Spleen/Kidney Yang Deficiency) — p. 131, 132
Indigestion (Phlegm-Damp) — p. 59, 113
Indigestion (sticky stools) — p. 51
Indigestion (undigested food) — p. 28, 39, 53, 89, 109
Initial dry and hard then soft and thinner stool — p. 37
Insomnia — p. 29, 61, 74, 83
Irregular or awareness of heartbeats — p. 67, 83
Irregular menstrual — p. 28, 35, 39, 48, 67, 83
Irritability and Restlessness — p. 31

J
Jaundice (yellow skin and eyes) — p. 110, 127
Joint and muscle pain — p. 99

K
Kidney Deficiency (bumpy stools) — p. 25
Kidney Deficiency (incontinence) — p. 131, 132
Kidney Deficiency (weak peristalsis) — p. 63, 134
Koilonychia/spoon-shaped nails — p. 45

L
Lactose intolerance (Dampness, Spleen Qi weakness) — p. 137
Leukorrhea — p. 39
Lightheaded — p. 45, 83, 127
Light yellow stool or watery stool — p. 19, 97
Liver Qi stagnation (green stool, stress-related stool changes) — p. 91
Loose stools (Cold-Damp) — p. 97
Loose stools (food allergies) — p. 77,
Loose stools (Qi Deficiency) — p. 63, 72, 91
Loss of appetite — p. 53, 59, 89, 127
Lower back pain — p. 28
Lipomas (lumps under the skin formed by phlegm and mucus) — p. 39, 72, 78

M
Malnutrition (thin/finger-like stool, Qi & Blood Deficiency) — p. 43
Menstrual irregularities — p. 28, 39, 46, 53,
Mental fatigue — p. 28, 39, 45, 53, 59, 67, 72
Mucus in stool (Dampness, Spleen Qi weakness) — p. 59, 113
Muscle stiffness — p. 97, 110
Muscle weakness — p. 28, 39, 45, 53, 59, 67, 72
Mushy stools (Liver–Spleen disharmony, Qi stagnation) — p. 51

N
Nail brittle — p. 41
Nausea — p. 59, 89, 104, 110, 122, 127
Night sweats — p. 29
Normal stool (color, shape, frequency) — p. 10, 11
Numbness and tingling — p. 74, 83
Nutritional deficiencies — p. 53, 59
Nutritional therapy (balance yin-yang, Spleen support) — p. 141, 142

O
Odors (stool fishy smells, Cold-Damp) — p. 13, 97
Odors (stool foul smells, Damp-Heat) — p. 13, 93, 122
Odors (stool sour smells, Spleen Qi Deficiency) — p. 13, 37, 63, 71, 119
Odors (stool rotten smells, overeating, food stagnation, food poisoning) — p. 13, 87

P

Painful bowel movements — p. 115
Pale complexion — p. 40, 67, 82
Pale lips — p. 67, 82, 127
Pale nails — p. 67, 82, 127
Pale skin — p. 45, 122, 127
Pale stool (Gallbladder or Liver Qi issues, bile obstruction) — p. 20, 107
Pale tongue with white coating — p. 40
Pale urine — p. 36
Pallor — p. 28
Palpitations — p. 67, 83
Parasites (worms, white dots in stool) — p. 57
Phlegm in stool — p. 65, 103
Poop chart (TCM stool analysis) — p. 147, 148
Poor appetite — p. 39, 61, 73, 79, 88, 92, 109, 122
Poor concentration — p. 28, 59, 78
Poor memory — p. 28, 67, 74, 83
Post nasal drip — p. 78
Prebiotics — p. 139
Prefer cold drink — p. 35, 94
Preference for cold environments — p. 35
Prefer hot drink — p. 39
Preference for warm environments — p. 39
Premature ejaculation — p. 28
Premature graying hair — p. 29
Probiotics — p. 139
Prolapse, sagging organs (hernia, anus, uterus prolapse) — p. 39, 65, 132
Prolonged bleeding from minor injuries or cuts — p. 39
Prolonged recovery — p. 46, 73

Q

Qi (five major types) — p. 66
Qi Deficiency (fatigue, loose stools, incomplete evacuation) — p. 57
Qi stagnation (straining to pass stool, gas, burping) — p. 33, 39, 57, 64, 72

R

Rectal (itching, irritation, pain or discomfort) — p. 53
Red stools (bleeding, Liver Heat, hemorrhoids) — p. 21, 113, 125
Red tongue with yellow coating — p. 35
Redness face — p. 35
Reduced appetite — p. 67, 82, 104
Reproductive issues — p. 25, 39, 53
Respiratory issues — p. 59
Restless sleep — p. 93, 105

S

Sallow complexion — p. 53
Sensitivity to humidity — p. 88
Scanty menstruation — p. 67, 83
Shortness of breath — p. 67, 83, 122
Sink and sticky stools (Dampness blocking the Spleen) — p. 77
Sinus — p. 78
Skin Issues (acne, hives, rashes or eczema) — p. 31, 53, 59, 95, 105
Sleep disturbances — p. 53, 59, 110
Sluggish — p. 39, 78, 89, 94
Soft blobs stools requiring straining (Qi & Blood Deficiency) — p. 63

Sores on the lips — p. 35
Sour taste — p. 53
Spleen Qi Deficiency (loose stools, fatigue, Dampness) — p. 37, 43, 63, 71, 81, 119
Stomach Heat (dry, cracked stools, foul odor) — p. 28
Stool changes (color, consistency, odor) — p. 59, 89, 115
Stool shape (normal) — p. 11
Stress (Liver Qi stagnation, IBS) — p. 53
Strong-smelling — p. 83
Sugar (Dampness, mucus or fat formation) — p. 31, 41, 48, 55, 61, 69, 75, 79, 85, 91, 96, 106, 111, 116, 124, 129, 135, 137
Susceptibility to illness — p. 67
Swelling (ankles and feet) — p. 46
Swelling (lower limbs) — p. 28, 95
Swelling in the legs or ankles — p. 72, 78, 127

T
Taste changes — p. 53, 89, 110
Textures of stool (diagnostic meanings) — p. 11, 12
TCM organ clock (bowel movement timing) — p. 8, 9
Thinner hair — p. 29
Thirst and dry mouth — p. 35, 94
Tinnitus and hearing problems — p. 28, 83
Tongue (coated) — p. 79, 104
Tongue (dry and cracked) — p. 83
Tongue (greasy coating) — p. 78, 89, 95
Tongue (pale) — p. 36, 67
Tongue (red with yellow coating) — p. 35
Tongue (thick greasy yellow coating) — p. 95
Tongue (white or yellow coating with areas of pale discoloration) — p. 53

U
Ulcers — p. 46, 122
Undigested food in stool (Spleen Qi Deficiency, Cold-Damp) — p. 28, 39, 53, 89, 109
Urgent or loose stools — p. 104
Urine changes (strong smell) — p. 95

V
Vegetables (cooked vs raw) — p. 30, 139
Visible abdominal veins — p. 127
Vomiting — p. 59, 89, 110, 122

W
Water retention — p. 28
Watery stool (Cold-Damp) — p. 97
Watery stool (Damp-Heat) — p. 93
Watery stool (toxic) — p. 87
Weakness (muscle, knee or legs) — p. 28, 45, 67, 72, 122, 127
Weakened immunity — p. 39, 46, 72
Weight gain — p. 39, 72
Weight loss (unintended) — p. 45, 59, 115
Wheezing – p. 59
White worms/dots (parasites, Dampness) — p. 57

Y
Yang Deficiency (cold digestion, incontinence, sluggish digestion) — p. 34, 38, 97, 108
Yin Deficiency (dry stools, thirst, internal heat) — p. 29, 121, 134,
Yellowing of the skin and eyes — p. 110, 127

About Catherine Yung

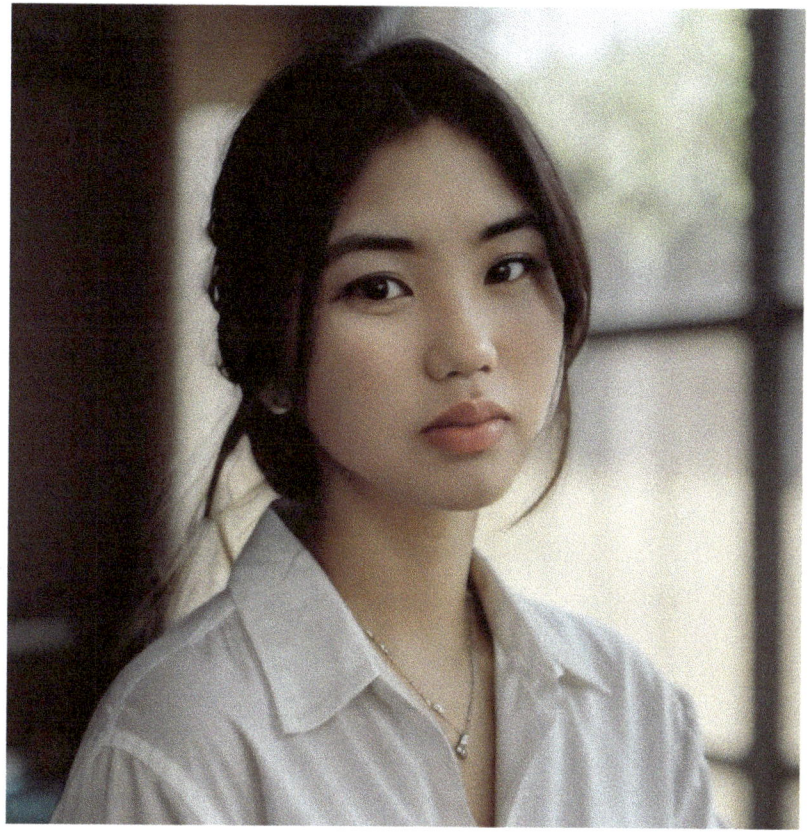

Catherine Yung is the daughter of herbalist Ann and the reason this journey into digestive health began. Born with severe gastric reflux and seizures, Catherine struggled early in life with what Traditional Chinese Medicine recognizes as a sensitive, allergy-prone body type — one especially vulnerable to external factors, poor digestion, and internal imbalance.

While Western medicine offered temporary relief, true healing came through generations-old herbal formulas and food therapy passed down in her family. Her full recovery sparked a deep respect for the power of natural medicine and shaped her lifelong commitment to holistic health.

Today, Catherine brings both lived experience and a modern voice to the ancient wisdom of TCM. She works alongside her mother to develop Silkie's herbal formulas, manage projects, and translate complex concepts into practical daily habits — especially around gut health and its most obvious indicator: your poop. She also oversees Silkie's social media and marketing, helping connect their family's herbal knowledge with a wider audience in fresh and accessible ways.

From her own healing to guiding others in understanding their body through stool patterns, Catherine is passionate about showing people how to restore balance naturally, especially those with sensitive constitutions like hers. Because when your digestion is right, everything else flows a little better.

About Patricia Nguyen

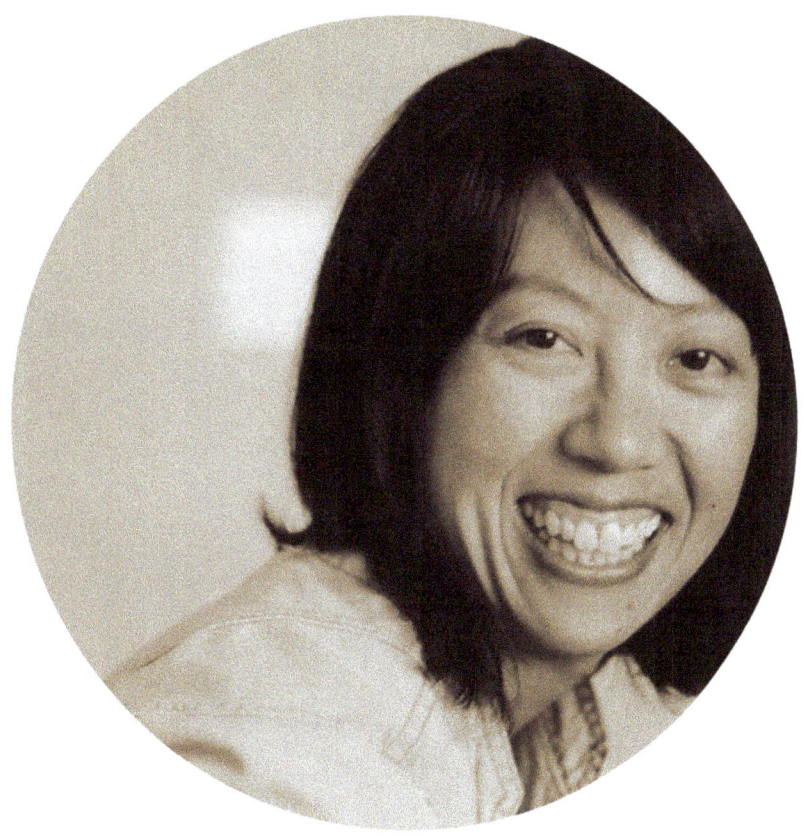

Dr. Patricia Nguyen, DACM, L.Ac., is a Doctor of Acupuncture and Chinese Medicine with over a decade of clinical and teaching experience. She maintains a thriving private practice in San Diego County, California, where she has helped hundreds of patients improve their health through the principles of Traditional Chinese Medicine (TCM).

Dr. Nguyen holds a B.A. in Asian Languages and Civilizations from Amherst College (1998), a Master's in Traditional Oriental Medicine (2013), and a Doctorate in Acupuncture and Chinese Medicine (2018) from the Pacific College of Oriental Medicine. She trained directly under Ann Tam, learning advanced herbal diagnostic methods rooted in classical TCM. Her specialties include digestive disorders, stress-related conditions, hormonal imbalances, chronic pain, autoimmune diseases, and emotional health.

Recipient of the Golden Flower Award in Herbal Medicine (2013), Dr. Nguyen is recognized for her excellence in herbal formulation and patient care. She also teaches continuing education courses for acupuncturists through Course Plus California CEU, helping practitioners refine their diagnostic and herbal skills.

Known for her compassionate and results-oriented approach, Dr. Nguyen empowers her patients to restore balance physically, mentally, and spiritually. When she's not in the clinic or classroom, she enjoys writing, mentoring, and her favorite hobby — pickleball.

About Ann Tam

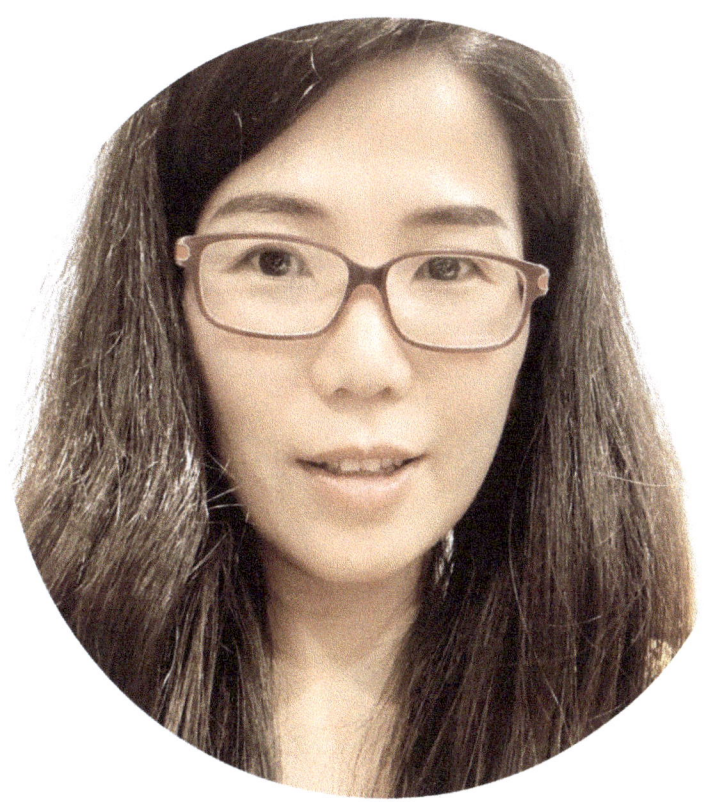

Ann is a fifth-generation herbalist whose lineage of Traditional Chinese Medicine practitioners stretches back to Imperial China. Born in Vietnam and raised in her father's herbal shop, Ann learned the foundations of herbal medicine from a young age — reciting herbal songs, identifying raw herbs, and helping prepare formulas. Though she initially walked away from the family trade, life had other plans.

After her second daughter suffered from severe gastric reflux and seizures, Ann saw firsthand the limitations of conventional medicine. In desperation, she returned to her roots. Under her father's guidance and with the help of family formulas refined over generations, her daughter made a full recovery — without the need for pharmaceuticals. That moment changed everything.

Ann dedicated herself fully to the practice of TCM, went on to study the medicinal benefits of natural plants at the University for Traditional Chinese Medicine and trained directly under her father and studied the ancient handwritten texts and medicinal records passed down by their ancestors. Through years of practice and observation, she came to deeply appreciate how much our digestive health - and especially our stool - reveals about the state of the entire body.

In Traditional Chinese Medicine, **poop is not just waste — it's a diagnostic goldmine.** Ann teaches that bowel movements are one of the clearest windows into internal balance, organ function, diet suitability, and even emotional health. This book is a result of her deep expertise and her mission to help people listen to their bodies through what they flush away each day.

Through her work at **Silkie**, Ann continues her family's legacy — formulating herbal supplements with only the highest-quality herbs harvested at peak potency, prepared with natural honey, and never containing fillers or synthetic ingredients. Every product is rooted in tradition and made with the same care her great-great-grandfather would have used.

This book is not just about digestion. It's about reclaiming the ancient wisdom of TCM to understand your health in the most natural, grounded way — starting with your daily poop.

Coming Soon

Recipes and Meal Plans for Different Body Types and Health Conditions

Your body's needs change with your constitution and health condition. In this upcoming book, you'll learn how to eat according to your body type — whether Hot, Cold, Damp, Dry, or Deficient — and support balance through food therapy based on Traditional Chinese Medicine.

Beyond body types, this guide includes specialized meal plans and recipes for common conditions such as:

High Blood Pressure — foods that calm Liver Yang and nourish Yin

High Glucose Levels — recipes that strengthen the Spleen and regulate Qi

Gout — dishes that clear Damp-Heat and support Kidney health

Skin Disorders — meals that cool Blood, expel Wind, and nourish the skin from within

Because we are what we eat, every bite matters. The right meal can heal — restoring energy, harmony, and balance from the inside out. Each recipe blends modern nutrition with generations of herbal wisdom to help you build lasting health, one dish at a time.

Stay tuned for updates and preorders at SilkieHerbs.com or follow us on:
Instagram: @SilkieHerbs
Ticktok.com/@SilkieHerbs
YouTube: Silkie Herbs Channel

THE POOP BOOK (VIETNAMESE)

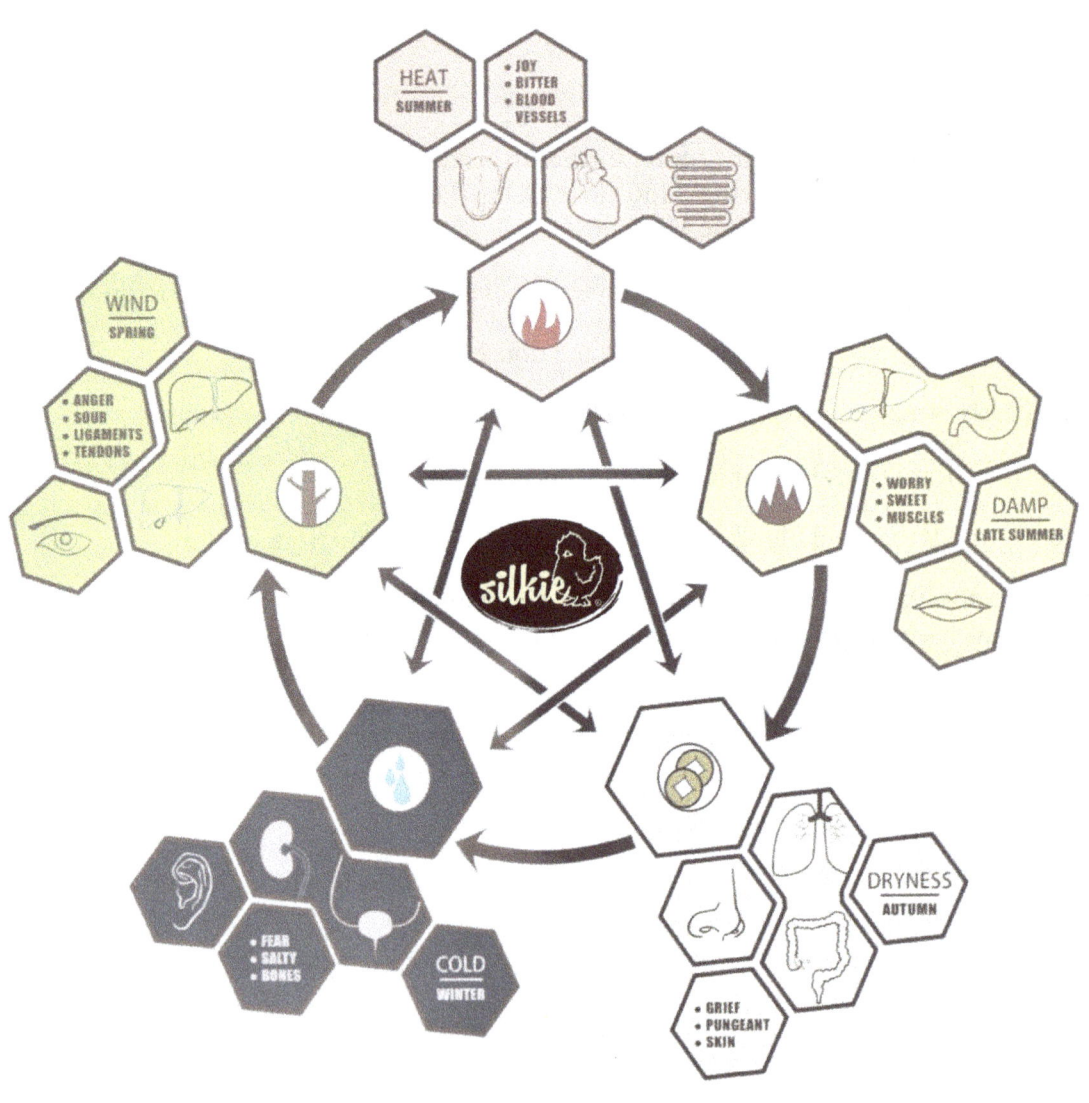

www.ingramcontent.com/pod-product-compliance
Lightning Source LLC
Chambersburg PA
CBHW080554030426
42337CB00024B/4868